BILLY

One Family's Insane Journey through the Virginia Mental Health System

Woody Hawthorne

chipmunkapublishing
the mental health publisher
empowering people with ADHD

Woody Hawthorne

All rights reserved, no part of this publication may be reproduced by any means, electronic, mechanical photocopying, documentary, film or in any other format without prior written permission of the publisher.

> Published by
> Chipmunkapublishing
> PO Box 6872
> Brentwood
> Essex CM13 1ZT
> United Kingdom

http://www.chipmunkapublishing.com

Copyright © Woody Hawthorne 2009

Chipmunkapublishing gratefully acknowledge the support of Arts Council England.

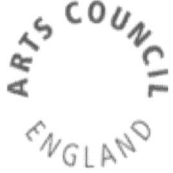

BILLY

Dedicated to my wife Janice, who without whose help our son would not have survived a single crisis

Woody Hawthorne

BILLY

Diagnosed with severe ADHD and bipolar disorder, Billy Hawthorne faced a steep uphill battle to control his mental illness and beat his debilitating addictions to alcohol and DXM products, the active ingredient in cough syrups such as Robotussin and Corocidin. Today Billy is managing his mental illness and his addictions and is ready to move on with his life, but not before relentlessly battling a crazy mental health and criminal justice system in Virginia whose plethora of contradicting rules and criteria many times came close to leaving him for dead.

Relive Billy's 5 year battle through repeated struggles and his ultimate triumph firsthand through the eyes of his father, Woody. It is both Woody and Billy's hope that, through reading this book, other families may be able to avoid much of the pain and craziness that kept Billy from getting better sooner.

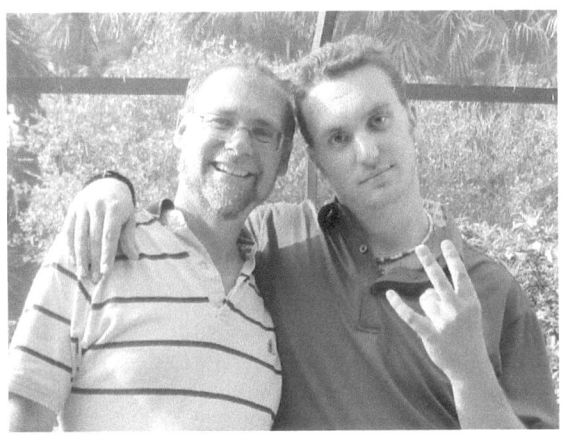

Chapter 1

It was just a typical hot day in July when my wife Janice felt the labor pains. The baby was coming early it looked like. Her water broke and she gave me a call at the office- time to get to St Lukes hospital in Cedar Rapids Iowa pronto. My coworkers at Rockwell Collins knew the call would come soon, but no one thought the baby was coming in July.

Exactly a year earlier Janice had surgery to have a baby. She had had her tubes permanently tied 9 years earlier after three children with her first husband, and never expected to have any more. That all changed when we got together in 1981 in King George, VA, we knew we were going to get married and we both wanted to have a baby together. We even independently came up with the baby's sex and name- we would have a girl named Sara. Problem was reversing the procedure was very new, and chances of it being successful were not so good then. The doctors told us the surgery would be like trying to sew two hollow hairs together on the outside while leaving the inside open. Just after we got married we had a consultation with the doctor who initially gave us only a 15% chance of having a baby together. That was depressing- we wondered if we should even keep pursuing this dream of ours. We did anyway and to our surprise, each test we did was a bit more encouraging than the last. It turned her tubes were only burned, and that made them easier to repair. Finally the odds were good enough to do the surgery (insurance paid the entire bill back then) so on July 27 1982 she went under the knife. The surgeon, Doctor William Davis, or "Wild Bill" as the nursing staff knew him, came out of the operating room with good news- the surgery went very well and we now had an 80%

BILLY

chance of having a baby. A big turnaround from the 15% number we heard 4 months earlier!

Despite being warned of the hundreds of things that could go wrong, we felt like God was smiling down on us in December when at the bottom of that pregnancy test tube was a big ring. We cheered- and then froze the test tube for posterity, and it was later found by the three girls who moved into the rental house after we had left.

When Janice was 7 months along, she brought up something we both had in the back of our minds- what if our Sara Jane turned out to be a boy? We had had an ultrasound done at 6 weeks, with inconclusive results. We both felt like we did not want to have another ultrasound and spoil the surprise, but at this point we were both really curious. We both agreed that the doctor had done miraculous work repairing those fallopian tubes (nationwide at that time less than 50% of couples who had this procedure conceived a child) that we would name the baby William Davis Hawthorne if it was a boy.

On July 26, 1983, contractions started coming faster as the day turned to night. We had practiced for this day for months in Lamaze class, but things did not go completely according to plan. They told me if Janice was not listening to the breathing instructions to just get in her face. It didn't matter- the pain was bad and there was some screaming going on. The time between contractions seemed to peak at 3 minutes around 10 pm, but then they just seemed to stop. The doctors felt that the baby should be delivered within 12 hours of the water breaking, so they gave her Pitocin to get the contractions going again. Boy did it work. After just 30 minutes Janice told the nurses the baby was coming-they scoffed and told her it would be another 30 minutes before the Pitocin would take effect. She insisted this was her body and she knew when a baby was coming. Suddenly the nurses were telling everyone to get organized and the table broke away into a birthing bed. I was thrown a blue smock and the show got on the road quickly.

All the way to the last second I thought that a girl was going to pop out, but alas it was indeed a boy. A very handsome healthy boy. It was a thrill to get the chance to cut the cord. He had swallowed a lot of fluid during the birth so they wisked him straight to intensive care. Janice didn't like the fact that other babies in intensive care had toys so she snuck down to the gift shop on the first floor and bought Billy his first toy- a plush Shamu. He was born at 8 lb 1 oz even though he lost a few ounces in the incubator over the next few days, he stabilized and a week later they let us take him home so long as we agreed to take him back for a few more blood checks- we happily agreed. I still remember listening to John Lennon's "Beautiful Boy" on the stereo when we got back to our Marion, IA home.

Billy came home to a big reception- our homey Iowa neighborhood spoiled us rotten and everyone wanted a look at the baby. We didn't have to worry about dinners for a week, and the baby gifts kept on coming. We brought Lisa and Eric back from the summer visit with their father early so they could see the baby. Our "miracle baby" was fitting right in and we could not be happier.

BILLY

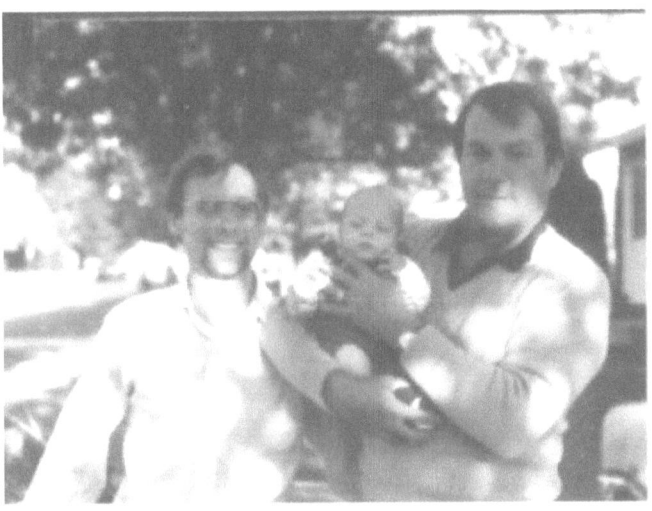

Here I am with baby Billy and my father Carlton in Marion, IA in September 1983. Billy was the only grandchild he lived to see- boy was he proud!

Billy grew up fast- at 6 months he was crawling, and he took his first steps on my first day at Harris Corporation in Melbourne, FL at just shy of 11 months. He seemed to be free from the "wet lung" that sent him to the hospital numerous times, and now he was filled with curiosity and laughter like any other child his age.

The following four years Billy was really fun to be around. He had a great prowess for the water at 3 years old, and could dive for quarters in a regular sized pool as long as you would throw them. Once he figured out he wouldn't drown if he put his head under water, he became a little fish. He also loved video games, especially donkey kong. He managed to play 2 years of T-ball in Palm Bay. He was full of energy but also very smart with an above average IQ. He was taking the bedtime story books to read himself at age 4. Any regrets that we had by not having a "Sara" quickly passed- Billy became the light of our lives.

BILLY

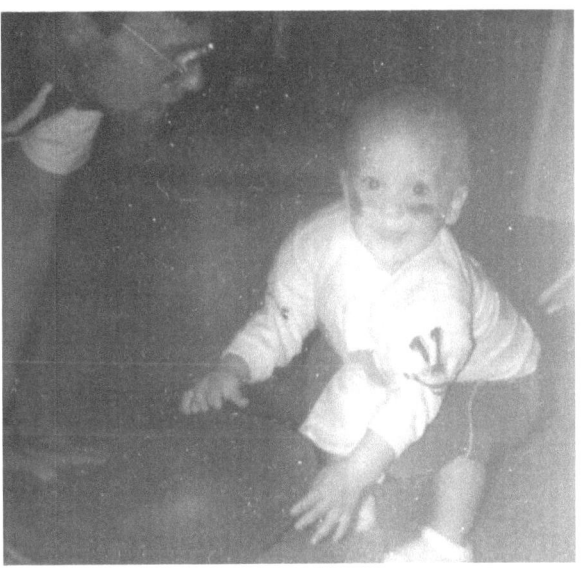

Billy dressed up for Halloween in October 1984- I think he was ready to recover a fumble!

Chapter 2

Billy always seemed full of energy growing up- he would run around the living room until he dropped, he loved racing to the fence and had to work to stay still long enough in the outfield make a catch. Still, I thought he was just energetic kid- he was always happy and inquisitive. One of our favorite memories is when the song "We are the World" came out in support of the starving people of Africa, Billy grabbed a pair of sunglasses, put them on upside down, and ran out in the living room in nothing but a pajama top to sing "We are world, we are chil-den" and wave his head around like Stevie Wonder. He was pretty well behaved in kindergarten, and was always happy.

BILLY

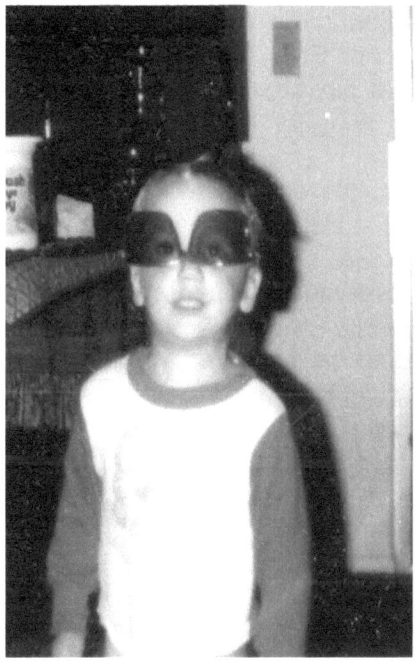

Billy doing his best "Stevie" imitation in May 1985- we are world, we are chil-den!

Woody Hawthorne

Billy started kindergarten just after he turned 5 at Port Malabar Elementary in Palm Bay, FL. As the fall went on we noticed he had a little more "Pelican power" than usual, and had a hard time listening to the teacher. This was especially true when he had the attention of the other kids. The problem came to a head when his teacher Ms. Parks called home in tears – it seems that Billy had jumped on top of the desk in the middle of class and did an "Elvis the Pelvis" dance. Nothing the teacher did that day seemed to help- timeouts, scolding nothing.

We were all perplexed. I was noticing the same thing when we were playing together. Billy would get into a silly zone and just start dancing or hollering or singing and the fact everyone stopped and stared at him didn't change anything. Again, if he heard even the slightest giggle he would be bolstered. Soon he was running where he was not supposed to and saying inappropriate things constantly, and I got used to chasing him down when he would disobey a rule then run. He would curse the fact that his Dad was a track runner, but catching him and punishing him constantly got old fast.

By second grade, we noticed his out-of-control behavior seemed to be worse in the afternoon, so in the second half of the year we just decided to bring him home at lunch and keep him home. Although the teachers were very appreciative, the school board told us that we were doing this "without their approval". Janice and I set up our own activities for him in the afternoon, and allowed plenty of outlet time. One memorable activity was taking him to a tax client of mine to look at all of the masks from her trip to Africa. The school tested him and found he had Attention Deficit Hyperactive Disorder (ADHD) and on the last day of school let us know his afternoon absences were "approved". Glad we didn't

BILLY

wait for the go ahead before we did something…. Little did we know this would be a portent of things to come.

Billy made it through kindergarten, but the school noted that Billy was not mature enough to be promoted to first grade. They recommended he go to Transitional Kindergarten instead. We were a little miffed at this assessment at first, but his teacher insisted that Billy would do better if it took it slower. Reluctantly we agreed, only to have that same teacher THEN recommend he repeat kindergarten (obviously TK classes were full). We refused and it was on to TK.

We took Billy in to see our own doctor where he was diagnosed with ADHD. Now what? And .. was that the only thing wrong with him? The doctor let us know there was a new wonder drug available for Attention Deficit Disorder (ADD) and ADHD called Ritalin. Ritalin is a stimulant when taken by persons without ADD, but for ADD patients it has an amazing calming effect. Cautiously we tried him on a small dose first and indeed he seemed to be calmer and think clearer! Finally we were getting a full school day out of Billy and it was great.

But the benefits did not come without side effects. He was not eating as well as he did and he actually lost some weight. He was staying up later and it was harder to get him to go to sleep at night. But considering he was now able to concentrate and make it through school days, we were grateful for Ritalin. So was Ms. Walker.

When Billy was in fifth grade, his therapist recommended he see another psychiatrist. This psychiatrist had his "own" theory that Billy was suffering from "rapid birth syndrome", a syndrome he alone had identified (created). Since Billy had swallowed a lot of fluid during his birth, the psychiatrist postulated that this was the cause of Billy's hyperactivity. Although we had never heard of such a syndrome, the psychiatrist was convinced of its validity. He ordered us to immediately stop giving him Ritalin and take only all natural remedies (such as vitamins). Needless to say, Billy almost immediately returned to his out-of-control behavior in the classroom, and soon the teachers were calling us wondering what happened and threatening to expel Billy from school if things didn't improve soon. We stopped seeing The psychiatrist and Billy's therapist apologized for ever sending us to him. He returned to his regular dose of Ritalin and all was well again. We learned a big lesson about just taking a new psychiatrists' advice without asking a lot of hard questions and staying involved at all stages of Billy's therapy. If this was going to be something we had to deal with all through his adolescence (and possibly his whole life), we could not afford to treat his therapy casually. We learned to trust our instincts because when it all came down to his treatment, we suffered the consequences of any bad diagnosis or treatment, not them.

Armed with Ritalin, Billy kept his grade level all through elementary school. When his IQ was tested he scored a 139 with particular aptitude for reading and writing. Through this time period, Billy read constantly and was always interested in new words and books. He learned how to use the Macintosh computer with very little help, and I actually got 7 year old Billy to help Mom access a file she needed over the phone!

During this time my father-in-law Calvin Grady passed away. A WWII veteran under General Patton, it looked like all those years of smoking caught up with him I am afraid. He passed away in early 1994 despite a last

BILLY

chance try by Janice to save his life by having heart surgery in Tampa, FL General Hospital.

On the way up to his funeral in Arlington National Cemetery, my mother in law Ethel started to act very strangely. Apparently she had developed an addiction to pain pills, and on the way up to Arlington from Palm Bay, FL she was getting antsy because my wife made sure she only got her prescribed dose. We decided to stop in Savannah, GA for the night even though Ethel objected. When we stopped at a Comfort Inn and I was loading the suitcases upstairs, I looked back in the car to see Ethel trying to grab her pain pills and was actually punching Janice! I split them apart and called the police to see if we could have Ethel taken to a hospital for the night. To our amazement, the police took her to a local mental health evaluator who told us that despite what happened in the parking lot, Ethel looked "lucid" at that moment and "did not meet the criteria" to be taken into a hospital. My wife told the mental health evaluator that her mother tried to commit suicide via overdose 10 years earlier, but she was told was happened previously did not matter because she looked "lucid" at this moment! The discussion was abruptly ended when another patient tried to steal prescription medication while everyone was still in the room.

Frustrated, we had no choice but to bring her back to the hotel, but again she refused to come up to the room for the night. We and all the hotel guests were awaked at 7 am the next morning with Ethel leaning on the car horn. Again the police and ambulances were called, but they warned us there was little point in calling mental health because she would be deemed "lucid" and released. Desperate, I asked the police officer what were supposed to do- I was not going to travel anywhere with Ethel for fear she would lean out the window and scream to someone that we were abusing her! The officer begged me to take her to her North Carolina home and he gave us his card to use if she yelled at someone that we were abusing her. Sending her in an ambulance all the way to Elizabeth City, NC would cost $5000. Reluctantly we left our 9 and 19 year old sons in the hotel in Savannah by themselves so we could take Ethel back to her house in North Carolina. We missed the funeral and turned around and picked the boys up in Savannah and headed home where our hometown pastor Stuart Rowan had our own remembrance service for my father-in-law.

I remember thinking then- how could this mental health evaluator possibly declare Ethel of her right mind when clearly she hit Janice and threatened to do it again? And what was this time limit thing- so what if she looked "lucid" at that moment- she was out of her mind 30 minutes ago! Also- Ethel tried to commit suicide with those same pills 10 years ago- why on earth was that not relevant?

We all hoped that that nightmare was going to now be just a bad memory now that Ethel was back in North Carolina to stay. When we picked 9 year old Billy and 19 year old Eric up, we had no clue that the worst was yet to come.....

In 1994 I got the word that Harris Corporation was "right sizing", and although I was told I had done an exceptional job on our last project, I was informed that I was demoted to a level 3 and was taking a 6.5% pay cut. In 1994 management decided it had "too many chiefs" and not enough Indians to stay competitive, so the Government Systems Division cut pay and demoted employees who were not in software or systems engineering. I was one of many to get caught up in this

BILLY

new policy; some took 20% paycuts and were demoted two levels. It was a very depressing time, but when The Analytical Sciences Corporation (TASC) offered me a 32% raise from my old pay and a promotion to a higher grade level, I felt compelled to take it. Realizing their mistake, the management at Harris tried to keep me by lowering the pay cut to just 2 %, but noting they would not reinstate me as a level 4. So if I stayed, I would not get **any** pay raise unless I was promoted back to level 4, something they already said they were not going to do for a while (remember- we had too many chiefs and not enough Indians). I told them it was a nice gesture, but I was not going backwards and it looked like I was headed to Herndon, VA to start my career as a government consultant supporting the same contract as a government advocate (years later Harris actually admitted that what it had done in 1994 was wrong!).

I thought to myself- why is this happening? I am working a job I love with great people- I have just been told that my project could not have been completed successfully without me- and yet I was getting a demotion and a pay cut! That is so not fair! Sometimes in life things are not fair… a lesson that would turn out to help me make it through events that were to come later. At those times you need to take a deep breath, believe in yourself and find a way to carry on….

I later found out they advertised to replace my position with someone who was at my old level (level 4)… I never saw the sense in that. We all loved Florida, and I loved my job and who I was working with, but obviously management had a grand plan and I was just a small cog on a big wheel. On July 3, 1995, we packed up the house and left our home in Palm Bay, FL for TASC in Herndon, VA, hoping for better things to come.

Chapter 3

When we arrived in Sterling VA, a growing town 30 miles west of Washington, DC, we had heard the schools in Loudoun County, VA were good schools. Since Billy had been already tested in FL and found to be ADHD, we naturally assumed that we naturally assumed that he would qualify for special classes when he started sixth grade in Sterling Middle School. Wrong assumption. When we registered him for school we were told that Virginia schools did not accept test results from Florida schools, he would have to retake Virginia's tests to prove he was indeed ADHD. This meant that Billy would have to attend regular classes until the school got around to testing him. When they finally did that in November 1995, they found he was indeed ADHD (what a surprise!). Now we were told that Virginia schools offered no special accommodations to ADHD students. We reminded the principal that we understood that it was the law that schools accommodate every student with disabilities. She told us she had not heard of that law.

Needless to say we did not take her at her word. After we did a little research, we found that the Virginia Department of Education was obliged to accommodate any student with disabilities (including ADHD) under the Individuals with Disabilities Education Improvement Act of 2004 ("IDEA"), Section 504 of the Rehabilitation Act of 1973, the Americans with Disabilities Act, and other federal and Virginia laws and regulations applicable to the education of students with disabilities. By the end of the year when we did find an advocate and the principal was challenged, she claimed her failure to let us know the Virginia law was an "oversight". I guess the "oversight" served its purpose- they didn't need to dip

BILLY

into their purses to provide Billy any special accommodations that school year.

Before the next school year started, we planned to let the lease on our rental house expire and buy a house of our own in Sterling. The lease was up at the end of August 1996, so we called the landlord in June to let him know our intentions. The landlord told us he would rather we buy the house, we told him thanks but we weren't interested. We found a great house in Broad Run Farms and closed on it in mid August. To our surprise, the landlord informed us by letter that the lease was ongoing unless we formally sent him a letter 45 days in advance letting him know our intentions. In other words, we were now stuck renting the old house for ANOTHER month!

So we took extra special care to clean the house up from end to end. Despite this, we got a call from the landlord's agent that she had done an inspection without our knowledge while we were out of town, and determined that the damage to the house was extensive. Furthermore, she changed all the locks on the house despite the fact that we paid rent for the month of September! Sensing a rat, we called a lawyer to try to get our money back.
I stormed over to his house to demand a key with a police officer in tow and didn't get anywhere. He smugly told me to use my old key (??). A week later we received a huge bill in the mail for extensive damages, including the replacement cost for an entire downstairs carpet that was already 5 years old when we moved in! So, he was not returning ANY deposit and now demanding thousands more! For a couple who ALWAYS got their deposit back when we left a rental house, this seemed crazy. We found an attorney who was equally dismayed with the situation and took our

case just for a percentage of what he recovered. We took the bull by the horns and sued the landlord in court for our deposit back.

So in December 1996 it was off to court we went. Loudoun County was just getting its reputation for being the new "technology corridor" with AOL and others moving to the county, and the county's population was booming- leaving the county to continually play catch-up. Despite its tremendous growth, its court system was still rural. We would find that out soon enough. We were new to Virginia, while the landlord had lived in the county all his life.

We were in for a big surprise on December 16. Another couple was ahead of us, suing their landlord for their deposit back. They proved that the damage due to a hot tub overflow was there BEFORE they moved into the house, and the landlord did not dispute this. Despite this, the judge ordered the couple to pay for the damages done to the house BEFORE they moved in!

Despite this bad omen, we were next. We presented our case- how we worked for 3 days cleaning the house, we were locked out, how we honored the lease and how we were being asked to pay for things that wore out through normal wear and tear (like light bulbs). He even had the audacity to ask for damages for a toilet that was clogged 16 days after he locked us out of the house! We sent return receipted letters to his house; he refused to sign for any of them.

Despite this, the judge awarded ALL of the damages asked for without any justification. He added insult to injury by awarding him ALL of his legal fees! We appealed the decision and the judge set the appeal bond at $950.

BILLY

Before we knew what hit us, the landlord got a new attorney and immediately appealed the appeal bond! The circuit court judge awarded him a new appeal bond of over $2000, making pursuing the appeal an expensive proposition. We had our deposit taken from us, and now we were facing a high stakes game where there seemed to be no rules. I wrote the judge asking for an explanation, we wrote back that I would not be getting one.

We mulled over our options. If we had a trial in Circuit Court, we could ask for a jury. Certainly the jury would see the unfairness and reverse the ruling. But the more we asked about the process, we found how reluctant Circuit Court judges were to reverse rulings from their lower court buddies.

Just to cut our losses, we paid the judgment in accordance with our attorney's advice. Unfortunately he just paid the landlord the money and didn't get him to sign a letter releasing us of all further responsibility- a big mistake. The landlord waited a year, then demanded MORE money to cover his legal bills during the appeal! We had to get a NEW lawyer, one from Manassas, VA and not in any "good ol boy" network. She immediately pointed out that the landlord had three chances to protest the award and ask for more money but declined, and now it was too late to come back demanding more fees! I wrote the opposing attorney demanding an explanation and accounting for $2800 in fees involved in defending our appeal, he told us he would not give them to us. They assigned us the SAME judge in General District court to hear the case, but when I wrote a letter to him asking the opposing attorney to provide us a fee breakdown, he CALLED the attorney to told him to provide it to us (very strange!). Our attorney made a motion to dismiss the case because the landlord had plenty of chance to ask for those fees earlier and didn't, but again the judge ruled against us and we proceeded to trial.

Then we finally got a little break... the landlord's attorney forgot that he sent an accounting of his fees that only totaled $1400- which we were ready to throw back at him. He then threatened to declare a "no-case"- throw out everything- cancel the lawsuit and start a new one. At the 11th hour, he called our attorney ready to settle- which we did for $2000, not even enough to cover his current attorney bills. And this time- we got our signed letter releasing us of all further responsibility.

Our rental nightmare was finally over- almost 3 years later. It left us angry, befuddled and a lot lighter in the wallet. We realized if a judge ruled it, everyone took the decision as gospel whether it made sense or not. This was our first experience with the Loudoun County Courts... little did we know there would be many more encounters ahead.

BILLY

Chapter 4 - Middle School

As Billy progressed through middle school, his behavior gradually deteriorated. Now in addition to being hyperactive, he was getting increasingly moody and dark. At 13 he was talked into breaking into the local elementary school down the road by two older boys and had to serve community service and pay restitution. Gradually he lost interest in playing outside games with other boys and seemed to be getting quiet and moody more often. When not being a disruption at school, he would retreat to his room more and more. We saw less and less of his happy smile and more stubbornness and backtalk.

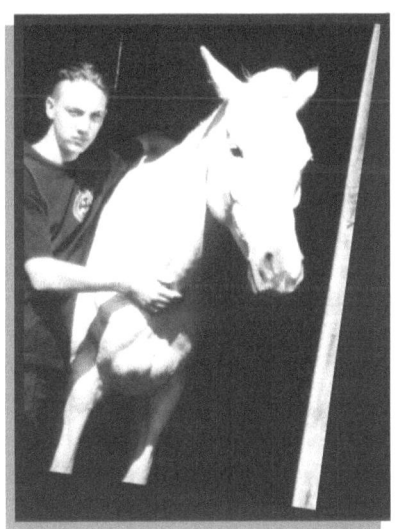

Billy horsing around in 1999

One trip we took we bought a bottle of wine (for us of course) and we stopped in at a restaurant for dinner on the way back home. We thought it was odd that Billy had to go back to the car in the middle of the meal. To our surprise we noticed the wine bottle was out and half of its contents were gone!

As problems with Billy continued, we realized we needed to take him to a therapist. We called our insurance company who recommended we go to a new psychologist because he was "in network" for our health insurance plan and we were given a limited number of sessions to start. Just like with the other therapists we consulted in Florida, I insisted that he set goals for Billy and we work toward them.

As the weeks went by, Billy seemed to getting worse. More moody, more angry and more resistant to seeing the psychologist. I really wanted to step in after the second session, but Janice urged me to give the psychologist a chance. Finally, after the fourth session ended with Billy angrily stomping to the car, I demanded to know what was happening at these sessions. the psychologist. had moved Billy into group therapy, and although Billy was only 13, he could not tell me anything about the sessions because of "client confidentiality". I told The psychologist.- he is 13 years old and he is getting worse for God's sake! In the same breath, The psychologist. tried to get me to have Billy sign up for another 7 sessions (part of the 11 preapprovals). I told the psychologist if he could not tell me anything about the sessions we would have to seek another therapist.

During this time Billy was also seeing a psychiatrist who recommended he move from Ritalin for his ADHD to Adderall as it came in a time release formula and did not have the same side effects as Ritalin (lack of appetite and trouble going to bed at night). The Adderall seemed to do better but the side effects were not completely

BILLY

gone. It was around this time Billy's mood continued to darken and he began associating with the "Goths" with their dark makeup and painted fingernails.

Billy was sinking deeper and we now needed another therapist – our insurance recommended another therapist in Leesburg. We asked our first the first psychologist to write an evaluation, and we were sorry we did that! Earlier in the year Billy had been attacked by the "wiggers" and school- the psychologist apparently thought Billy was talking about the "niggers" and wrote that Billy had a problem with other races! Furthermore, he wrote that Billy was now taking "Atoral" which prompted the new the psychologist to wonder who on earth was treating Billy.

As before, I pressed the new therapist to see if he could come up with a plan to help Billy after he evaluated him. Because Billy was still just 13, we didn't want to hear that consultations with him were "confidential". The therapist evaluated Billy for the minimum number of sessions then announced he would not treat Billy anymore because "only Billy could help Billy"

I thought- what in the hell does that mean? If "only Billy can help Billy", why are we paying this guy $125/hour? Do you get everyone's hopes up that you are going to help the boy, have us make all of our calls to insurance, take time off work so you can say "I don't feel like treating him anymore so see ya?" I asked if he reached an impasse with his treatment, he said no. I asked if he felt Billy was getting better, he said no. He was just going to stop treating him. His prerogative.

No follow-on recommendations, just a stupid ass philosophic statement that justified a therapist's laziness. I guess I mistakenly assumed there was some professional courtesy among therapists, psychologists and psychiatrists- like doctors. Here we were again- Billy was getting worse, and now the therapist just feels like quitting- so we get out the insurance list and try again.

Before we could do that, Billy had what looks like his first manic attack around the same time. His eyes got wide, he wanted to fight everyone, and he would not listen to anyone. We reluctantly took him to a mental hospital in Leesburg.

There we told that we were in a "borderline" situation. In Virginia, Billy had to give consent to be in a mental hospital unless he was kept there by a Temporary Detention Order (TDO). Amazingly, the nurse got 14-year old Billy to "agree" to stay at the hospital and be evaluated, but after the "agreement" he threw a tantrum in the hallway. The tantrum, surprisingly, didn't seem to help or hurt his case.

I thought why on earth does a 14 year old get to decide if he needs to go to a mental hospital when his parents are insisting that he be admitted... for good reason? I can't imagine too many circumstances where an out of control 14 year old would voluntarily agree to go to any hospital. What kind of rule was this? Was this there to protect the rights of a 14 year old? With an option like this given to him, he could just refuse and let a situation escalate out of control really quickly. I also noticed that it seemed to me that all the "professionals" seemed to buy into this rule whether it made any sense or not.

Billy was scared in his first visit to a mental hospital. He roomed with two guys with some real serious problems. Janice insisted we visit on a Friday of a 3 day stint and that proved to be a mistake- all he did was beg for us to

BILLY

let him out while promising to "be good". We allowed him to be released the next day, but the "honeymoon" while back at home was brief.

Later that year Billy was attacked from behind at his middle school, Farmwell Station in Ashburn, VA. A kid told another kid that Billy called him a racist name, and without inquiring further Billy was hit from behind by two kids a head taller than him. The principal suspended the two attackers, but claimed it was partially Billy's fault because he dressed oddly and invited the attack. Furious, we took the incident to the Loudoun County Police intake office. To me it was an open and shut case- the two boys were caught attacking Billy; they left a knot on his head- guilty! To our amazement, the intake officer seemed to do his best to justify not charging the boys with anything. He claimed that putting Billy on the witness stand to be questioned by lawyers would be "intimidating and scary" for Billy- maybe the best way to cope with the trauma would be for him to take karate(????). He also claimed that since Billy told the attacker "you didn't hurt me" after he was hit in the head, that it would be hard to get a conviction. I countered with the fact we had the boys caught in the act and a huge bruise on Billy's head- I think THAT was enough to get a conviction no matter what was SAID. In addition, the boys had ALREADY been found guilty at school and punished. We left the juvenile office very frustrated, because we thought that if they didn't charge the boys, we could not go forward. Why were they doing this? To reduce the number of court cases possibly?

We DID call the parents of the attackers and asked that they split the $96 medical bill we received for taking Billy to the doctor the day he was attacked. One parent agreed that the attack was barbaric and reimbursed us for their half of the medical bill and made the boy pay for it out of his pocket. We were glad to see a parent step up because the Loudoun County intake sure as not going to do it.

One positive development that happened while Billy was in Farmwell Station Middle School-we met an advocate of impaired students- Ms. Sharon Spinelli. Sharon had helped many other students get special allowances because of their handicap, and she fought hard with the administration at Farmwell Station to get Billy some allowances when he would act up (in terms of removal from the class) and got him the right to use a laptop to take notes as taking them longhand was killing his hands. In the midst of the craziness she was one of the angels. For all the work she did for us she refused to take a dime. Unfortunately he didn't take advantage of those allowances like he should have.

BILLY

Chapter 5- Juvenile Detention and Probation

As time passed, Billy's moodiness, darkness and anger continued to increase. While at a family outing at Urbanna, Billy got very mouthy and attacked me. I got him in a headlock on the street in front of my mother, sister, brother-in-law and brother just before dinner time and we had to leave to go home. The entire trip home he was screaming at us and I actually had to restrain him again in the car, causing my wife to pull over a couple of times.

After things had settled down, I tried to figure out what set him off. I talked to Billy later on and he just said he was mad and felt like fighting someone. From what I could tell it was totally unprovoked.

Billy's social life was changing too. He no longer had happy friends who liked to laugh and play video games, he seemed to only have friends who were into witchcraft or were "goth". He started wearing his hair over his eyes, putting on black makeup, wearing trenchcoats inside buildings and staring a lot at the wall. Over this time Billy continued to see therapists, although again I could not see where they were making any progress in determining what was wrong. Half of the therapists said he was bipolar, the other half said he was not. When I pressed one of the therapists on whether there was a test for bipolar, I was told no. Being bipolar meant Billy was both manic and depressed, and the criteria on what constituted mania and depression was blurry and subject to interpretation. This diagnosis proved important because the psychologists who thought he was bipolar gave him medication for that, and those that did not would only give him medication (Adderall) for his ADHD condition. The medications for these conditions can be opposed to each other. We saw tremendous mood shifts when Billy changed psychologists. Despite our pleas, we could not get a new psychologist to talk to a former psychologist. I assumed the new psychiatrist thought the old psychiatrist was totally off base with his diagnosis and Billy needed a radically new direction.

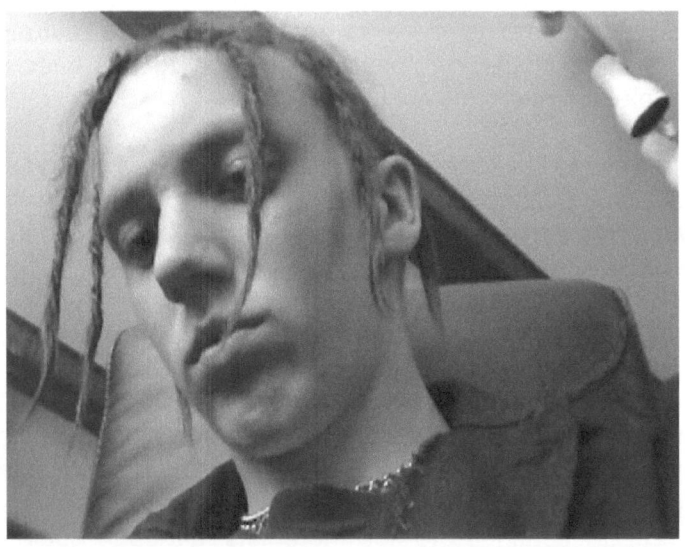

Billy (age 16) at the computer in 2000

The continual changes in therapists, psychiatrists and psychologists were due to many factors. Sometimes the number of visits allowed by our insurance company expired, sometimes Billy refused to see the psychiatrist again because after so many visits he didn't like him, or sometimes we could see that Billy was getting worse and HAD to have a change.

BILLY

Throughout this entire time, I was still mystified why it was so difficult to talk to a therapist or a psychologist about my 15-16 year old son. Despite my hope that we could observe his problems and team with doctors to find a solution for them, nothing seemed to be improving. I was told that the doctors and therapists didn't want to violate confidentiality laws. I told them Billy didn't say much of anything about their sessions, and I wouldn't expect a 15 year old with a mental illness to be very comprehensive about the session. Even when we got Billy to sign a release to so the therapists could talk with us, they typically would then let us know that talking to parents about a patient was not their style. How in the world are we supposed to help this young man if we can't know what the doctors are doing or not doing to try to help him? I was quickly getting the feeling that many were in business to collect their $150 - $200 per hour fee for as long as they could string us along then move on to other patients who had a new set of visit approvals.

As 9th grade was coming to a close, we realized Billy was about to fail physical education because he had missed so much time due to mononucleosis. The teacher was going to fail him for sure unless we could provide proof from the doctor that all the missed time was due to mononucleosis. We went to the doctor who certified that all of the time missed was due to illness, and after we submitted the paperwork, the teacher agreed to pass Billy but he had to attend her class every day until the end of school, which turned out to be 6 class days. After all of this effort, Billy greets us on Monday morning with "I am too tired to go to school". I told him that after all we did to keep him from failing this class; we would carry him into the class room if we needed to. I proceeded to pull a shirt over his tired head when he swung at me. Again I got him in a headlock and the police were called to the house.

When the police arrived, they pulled Billy from the headlock I had him in and calmed him down. Then, he called someone to check if they should bring ME in for domestic violence! They noted that normally if there is a domestic disturbance, Virginia law requires them to arrest someone for domestic violence. Since I was the adult, I would normally be considered the "bigger threat", whether I simply restrained Billy or not. And all this was up to the discretion of the officer. I quickly realized that Billy could start a fight with me at my own home, I would restrain him and I might be arrested for domestic violence. He may start 10 fights, if he could get one officer to arrest me, it could jeopardize my job. Crazy!!

Earlier in the month he had learned of all the "restrictions" that parents were under as far as treatment of their unruly teenagers as per Child Protective Services in Loudoun County VA. One of the rules was that we parents could not lock our teens out of the house when they were cussing at us or acting outrageous-this was considered "denial of domicile" and was a crime. Some of these rules seemed bent on giving the unruly teenager control of the household. Though he never did challenge these rules, I was ready to face charges before I let my out of control teenager rule my house.

The moods and the outbursts continued and seemed to culminate in September of 1999. While I was out of town on business, Billy had managed to get a hold of a lot of Peyote. He told Janice he was going to leave the house; she blocked his path and said there was no way he was leaving the house in that condition. He tried to

BILLY

push past her in the hallway and all hell broke loose. Our family picture came crashing down on both of them, and Janice grabbed Billy's hair. During the struggle, my stepdaughter Lisa called the police and the police actually pulled Billy off of his mom. While they were coming, Billy gave Lisa an evil laugh and told her "You better hurry and call them quick…"

This time the police arrested him and took him to jail. I got a call while on business in Florida and cancelled the rest of my trip to come home just in time for the hearing. Billy was assigned a court appointed attorney to defend him. The first thing he did was pump Janice and Lisa for information only to turn it around against us. When I got to court, Billy was trying to decide whether to have a trial or not- I talked to Billy and encouraged him to plead guilty- he DID hit his mother- and avoid forcing us to testify against him. The attorney advised him to go to trial so that's what we did. I had to take pictures of Janice's arm and we all testified against him… and that was painful. He was convicted of assault on his mother and was sentenced to 45 days at juvenile detention.

I did not know why Billy was acting this way. He had done Peyote and his older brother Eric noted that that substance stayed in your body a long time. Certainly it contributed but seemed to be a culmination of a gradual building of anger and craving for drugs.. any drugs that could not be quenched. Worse, it seemed with all the psychologists, therapists and psychiatrists Billy had seen and all the medication he had been prescribed those we were no closer to identifying much less solving his problems.

He was allowed to serve some of his time in a juvenile halfway house, which I actually think helped him. We missed seeing our Washington Redskins football team play but we visited him every Sunday and worked very hard to get his 10th grade homework sent to him at the juvenile facility. I first was told they would take care of it, but after a week they had yet to call the school. I called the school and made a pain of myself until the facility HAD to pick up his homework so he would not fall behind. Finally the facility director came to Billy and insisted that he do his homework so that his father (me) would leave him alone!

Billy had a particularly tough time in the juvenile detention center. We were told at that time that Loudoun had the BEST juvenile detention center in Virginia but the worst adult detention center in Virginia. When he would not follow an order he was ordered to solitary for 12 hours, where he screamed for his mom and ripped his clothes. It was very painful to see him escorted in to the juvenile halfway house in shackles… there were plenty of tears that night. Janice and I had hoped that Billy would straighten out when he got out of juvenile detention, but we knew that was not going to happen without a lot of help.

Billy was released from Juvenile Detention on Nov 8, 1999 with all kinds of probation. We had a chance to talk to him on Sundays and were convinced that he had no intentions of hurting his mom; he was just out of control that night. However it was looking like the number of times he was getting out of control was increasing and still we had no real reason why this was happening.

During this time Janice and I joined a support group that met weekly in Leesburg- Parents of troubled teens. This was a great support group that we got a lot from. Lots of great speakers and fellowship. The more we went we realized there were a lot of parents struggling

BILLY

to raise their kids without breaking the law. All of the group parents had to call the police to their house more than once when their child was out of control, and all had seen police responses from "We may need to arrest you for being the bigger threat" to "we are here to calm things down". In nearly every case, drugs were involved.

In February 2000 Billy was caught with marijuana in school and back to court he went. This time the juvenile court ordered US to take a parenting class from them called the Leadership Education Awareness for Parents (LEAP) Program. This daytime class was given by Community Corrections (responsible for juvenile probation). The class hours (mid day on a weekday once a week) were really awful and I think the department got a certain enjoyment in watching working parents struggle to get off work during prime time (9- 5 M-F) to attend this class. Unfortunately, the day of the first class I had to get my supervisors signature to get a key government clearance or I would not have been able to work the job that we had lobbied for over 6 months. My immediate supervisor refused to sign the request, noting that in his opinion my acoustic database project was going "nowhere". So I had to appeal to the director to get it done- and my appeal paid off. It was now or never- I got the signatures and got the paperwork to security before the end of the day and was now able to work the job.

I knew I had to take the LEAP class so I got the notes from Janice and took off work to attend class #2 of 6. To my shock, I was told there was an (unpublished) rule that no one could miss the first class for any reason. I could stay until the end of the class, but I would be given no credit. I checked the class brochure and there was no mention of the rule. I was told not to come to the third class.

Billy's court appointed attorney again turned out to be the same one he had earlier. After he pushed Billy to go to trial in October of 1999, I was none too pleased with him, but as Billy's attorney I had to be civil and talk to him. Later that week I told him about the craziness with the parenting class and he was incensed. He urged me to file a motion with the juvenile court to be able to take the class, and point out that NOWHERE on their list of rules was the requirement that the parent could not miss the first class for any reason. To me, the reason Corrections and the Court was so restrictive was to get deadbeat parents "off their butts" to parent their children, but the fact that it penalized other involved hardworking parents who found it very hard to get off work in the middle of the day was secondary. I followed his instructions on how to file a motion and faxed in copies to the court on a Thursday for a Friday hearing. Before they had a chance to cite me for anything, I was going to file a motion against THEM.

The next day at court there was a substitute judge from another county. Since I filed the motion, I pleaded to the court to allow me back in the class as missing the first class was unavoidable and I had made up the work the next day. The judge immediately announced that I "screwed up" by not showing up for the first class and dared me to respond. The prosecuting attorney wanted to find ME in contempt for missing that first LEAP class! I kept my mouth shut, but it was obvious that the judge was going to do everything he could to keep juvenile probation from looking bad. The head of the department who created the situation didn't even need to show up and the judge assumed the role as his advocate. After he realized that nowhere in the written

BILLY

rule was the "can't miss the first class for any reason" he ceased to allow me to speak. He then continued the case two weeks later so I would need to miss another day of work.

Two weeks later, the court appointed attorney volunteered his time to represent me free of charge. What a surprise! I was glad I didn't burn my bridges with him, because it looks like he came around to realize we were a good family who just wanted to save our son. When the prosecuting attorney saw that the public defender was voluntarily representing a citizen, he became incensed and that the public defender took over arguing the case for his representative. My little petition now became a heavyweight battle.

The public defender pointed out that we was entitled under Virginia statues to represent any one he wanted, and when the Judge could not find a way to deny the commonwealth attorney's objections, he turned to him like an old buddy, pulled off his glasses and said "Counselor, I am gonna have to say no this one". I had to gather evidence that I indeed had a legitimate reason for missing the class and had to have that same supervisor sign a sworn statement to that effect. I had to prepare well because if my case was not airtight, the judge was going to cite me with a failure to comply and fine me! When the root of the petition was finally addressed, the judge allowed me to repeat the class again penalty free at another time.

Before the petition concluded, the Judge looked at the very young and pretty representative from Juvenile probation and swooned, "And tell us about what good things you do". When the county attorney lost his petition argument, he suddenly accused me of being rude to this young and pretty representative on the phone! I thought I was cooked. Fortunately she was honest and fair and said I had in no way treated her rudely on the phone- phew! He might have jailed me if she said otherwise.

For all those police and corrections officers who advised me to just kick his ass and he would straighten out.. how crazy was this! I imagine this class was done this way to show a neglectful parent who was boss and to get off the stick and parent, but that model didn't fit us in any way shape or form. The class was interesting, but there was no mention on how we might handle a bi-polar child. In fact the subject of mental illness was not addressed at all. The theme of the class was- there are no bad children, only bad parenting. So if parents would parent better, there would be no bad children. Mental illness and chronic addictions did not fit into that model.

Billy was getting increasingly paranoid while at school. He barely finished 10th grade, and asked if he could do online school for 11th grade. Given the daily difficulties we had dealt with in 10th grade, I felt we didn't have much choice. We enrolled him in Alpha Omega Academy in September 2000.

It was around this time that Billy had his first experience with Robotussin cough syrup. Robutussin contains the active ingredient DXM, which if taken in high doses can cause some people to hallucinate. When huffing canned air and paint became boring, his "friend" thought he could get a Robotussin buddy if he introduced it to Billy. For 93% of the population, taking over the prescribed dose causes the ingestor to vomit violently. For those 7%, it is a cheap legal high that there is no test for. For those 7%, it was incredibly addictive.

BILLY

Even for the addict, he needs to not eat anything for a period of time to hold it down. According to Billy, he could see movies in "3D" when he was on it. Even as he became addicted to it, even he couldn't take it after he ate food or drank water. According to him he had to fast for days to be able drink bottles or swallow 32 to 64 Coricidin tablets.

In September 2000, we planned to take a cruise to Cozumel, Mexico and told Billy he could take a friend with him. The friend he chose, Richard, turned out to have a huge marijuana habit and he showed up at our house completely high in mid-September, so we refused to allow him to come (or see Billy again for that matter) despite the fact he had given us a big deposit. He later sold his ticket to Billy's girlfriend, Cindy who ended up going on the cruise in his place.

Billy's first Temporary Detention Order (TDO) occurred on November 8, 2000- election day. I stopped by Sterling Elementary to vote and got home around 6 pm. Billy was in a very belligerent mood and Janice and I followed the advice of the "class" and ignored him. He was wild eyed and high on something but we didn't know what. We then heard a lot of racket and had to see if he was breaking anything. We were horrified to see that he had put a huge steak knife to his chest and screamed that he was "really going to do it this time". We were smart enough not to rush at him, so we just tried to talk to him. Despite our pleas, he said he was working himself up to stab himself really good. Janice thought quickly and called his girlfriend Cindy and passed the phone to him. She managed to talk to him for a while, but ultimately he told her nothing mattered he was going to stab himself. He ordered me not to leave or he would stab himself, but I knew I had to try to do something. As Janice and Cindy talked to him I slowly inched out the front door and ran to the neighbors who called 911. The police were there in a flash, but when we got to the door we found the house filled with mace. Billy apparently had found the can of mace we had hidden, but aimed it the wrong way and sprayed himself. As he was coughing, Janice managed to talk him into letting go of the knife. With everyone coughing and eyes stinging, the police handcuffed Billy and took him to the police car. Strangely, all Billy could talk about was how he envisioned I was coming through a 2' x 1' window behind him to get him!

We were relieved that we somehow got to him before he had stabbed himself. Why on earth did he want to kill himself anyway? Why did he "see" me- 5'10" 170 lb man coming through a tiny window? We left the windows up to clear the house and headed to the hospital where hopefully Billy would get some help.

When we got to the hospital, we soon were talking to a Loudoun County Mental Health (LCMH) worker whose job it was to decide if Billy met the criteria for a TDO. They had Billy sedated in a hospital room as we talked. We had to go through the entire chain of events with the lady, who then talked to Billy. She came out and announced that Billy said he had smoked marijuana, and he had before. Then she looked at us with a long pregnant pause. I told her we were not aware of this and we certainly condemned its use in our house. The pause continued. I further told her that he must have worked hard to get it and do it secretly because while he was in the house we were always checking on him. I resented the fact that Billy's suicide attempt was being turned back on us!

Next we were told that in Virginia there was a four hour limit after a patient was taken in custody to either TDO

BILLY

someone otherwise they could be released. This seemed like a crazy law to us. It took an hour to interview us, more time to interview him and now we were coming down to the wire. After calling several mental hospitals, the LCMH worker came back to us and announced that she was having trouble finding a place that would take Billy and would we consider taking him back home.

"Are you crazy?" I asked. Why on earth would we take him home when he just tried to stab himself to death? So he could finish the job?

I asked the worker to keep trying and that we were absolutely NOT taking him home. After trying another two hospitals, she announced a facility in Richmond off of Janke Rd (Behavioral Health Services) would take him but that was the closest place she could get. I told her to accept it- I didn't care if it was in North Carolina!

Billy was treated and released 3 days later, and for a while we thought things were getting better. We were given an option to get him into an adolescent rehab program at that point, but at we felt it was too early to exercise that option. We had later determined that Billy had consumed 32 Corocidin tablets along with smoking marijuana and apparently that peaked his paranoia. We got a new therapist for him, a young lady just out of college who worked for the Loudoun County Mental Health auxiliary that was just across the creek from us in Sterling. We had hoped Billy could relate better to her and maybe open up to her on why he felt he wanted to kill himself.

Midway through December 2000, Billy ran away from home. He left a message that he was in a safe place, but he was not coming home. I traced a call we got in the middle of the day to a nearby grocery store, but he was gone by the time I got there. I posted flyers that we had a missing child in the area. Days later we got a call from a Reston mall, I drove down to the mall and found people who had seen him. By this time we had a cell phone to communicate. We gave up that night, and the next night found him at his girlfriend Cindy's apartment. We talked for a while and eventually got him back home in time for Christmas.

The peace was short lived however. As you might imagine, through all the TDOs and running away from home, Billy was well behind in his school work. On New Year's day 2001, I told him there was no TV until he got his homework done. He went for the TV remote anyway, I blocked his path and a full scale wrestling match was on. Again I was restraining him but I was mindful that if the Police were called they could rule that I was the "bigger threat" and arrest me for domestic violence. We managed to tie him up with ties, but we knew good and well he didn't meet TDO criteria. We knew that Behavioral Health Services in Richmond told us ANYTIME he was out of control they would take him so we put him in the car and headed south. On the way down Route 28 he was screaming, pulling Janice's hair and threatening to kill us. Finally when we reached Manassas he calmed down, cried and apologized. Not being sure that the mental hospital in Richmond would even take Billy, we turned around and went home. Later that week his therapist noted that threatening to murder your parents was "bad"-I think the problem was way over her head. Fortunately, my stepdaughter Lisa and her husband Todd asked if Billy wanted to stay with them in New Llano, LA and help take care of their son Christopher, and Billy agreed that was a good idea. Exhausted and exasperated, we sent Billy to his older

BILLY

sister's house and hoped for the best while we caught our breath.

Chapter 6

Janice and I got a temporary respite from the madness in January 2001 when Billy left to be with his older sister and her family for a few months. The peace was nice but we were constantly worrying how he was. He was enrolled in Alpha Omega home school but it seemed to take forever to get him back online to resume his studies. I found it hard to believe that my step daughter spent her fair share online with her chat friends and Billy could not seem to spend anytime getting his connection to the school. Billy spent his time watching his nephew Chris but without his Mom or Dad there, there just was not a lot of push to have himself keep up with his school work or avoid alcohol.

By March I had a long trip scheduled to support an EMI test at Harris in Melbourne, FL. We had hoped that staying with his sister would help him, but he did not seem to be getting better. It did give us a much needed break to recharge our batteries however. We decided that if Billy wanted to come back home he would have to ask to come home. He admitted he was ready to come home in March and Janice rented a car to pick him up in New Llano, LA and then meet me in Melbourne.

Soon after we got back to Virginia Billy again seemed to again be sinking back to darkness. He resumed his school work with Alpha Omega, but he was staying up all night and sleeping in the day. He had one friend, Tee, who he spent all his time with. Tee had dropped out of school and his father was a known marijuana user, so obviously this concerned us. For his 18th birthday in July he brought Tee to our time share in Williamsburg, VA and we hardly saw either one of them. They both slept until 3 in the afternoon every day... I

BILLY

was inclined to allow him to sleep during our vacation but found that I actually had to wake him up on his 18th birthday for his 6 pm party!!

During this time it is fair to say we were concerned with Billy's odd behavior, but since he was keeping up with his school work and staying out of trouble, we sort of reluctantly tolerated it. We took a trip to New York City in December that went without incident, but when we went to Galveston in February 2002 to visit my Uncle Cliff and family, Billy refused to get in the car that day because he had a "premonition we were going to crash." When we got to Galveston and went to the Houston Rodeo, all seemed ok until we were ready to leave and found a marijuana pipe. We disposed of it, but when Billy found out, he climbed up in the children's monkey bars and refused to leave until he got his pipe back. We had a stand off for 4 hours at the timeshare but we didn't budge-we told him at the very least bringing drug paraphernalia on the Army base at New Llano (we were staying with Lisa after the vacation) would get our son-in-law Todd in trouble. Again we were considering leaving him behind because he refusing to travel.

The "refusing to travel" trick particularly incensed me. As with most travel situations, advance plans needed to be made and advance tickets needed to be purchased. Billy tried to get his way by "refusing to travel" at the last minute and ruin the trip for the entire family. Many times he had hoped that we would just go without him and leave him at home to do drugs, but we were never going to let that happen. His actions cancelled a few trips, moving me to make travel plans by CAR only and to purchase insurance for timeshare reservations. Also, we made sure there were plenty of negative consequences for pulling that trick- like cutting out all rides to friends houses and cutting off video games.

We finally got home and again saw no real improvement. Billy's paranoia seemed to still be worsening, and drug incidents seem to be increasing. We had a few fun moments together, but those times were getting few and far between. In April and May 2002 his friends almost left him at music festivals because he was so strung out on drugs. These all turned out to be warnings of what was to come in June of 2002.

BILLY

Chapter 7

Saturday June 8 2002 started out like any other summer day around our house, except today we had the Northrop Grumman picnic at Smokey Glen Barbequers in Gaithersburg, MD. Traditionally this was an awesome picnic, with great food, fun sports and an all around great time. Janice had to work so she encouraged me to get Billy to go with me before he got into something. She went to work but as usual he was out until the afternoon and I knew all the food would be gone by then- so I left for the picnic. I could not live my life babysitting a sleeping teenager. I had a great time at the picnic and got to play some softball and eat ice cream cones. When I got home Billy asked what he could get me for father's day which was two weeks away and I told him I would love it if he could just stay awake enough to play catch with me for Father's day. So without saying another word he got the other softball glove and started tossing the ball- it was great!

Janice and I went to bed at our normal time only to be woken up at 4 am by a crazed Billy who was running around the house ranting that his girlfriend Cindy was sick- he just knew it- and he had to get to her house to save her. I told him it was 4 in the morning and we were not going anywhere. He asked me if he could ride MY bike over there and I told him no way... he was not going to lose MY bike along with the others he lost over the years. So he jumped on another bike and sped off- we were both too exhausted to pursue him.

We were again awoken at 6 am by Billy again demanding that we take him to his girlfriend's house so he could save her. I told him to calm down, I am sure she was fine and we were not driving him anywhere at the crack of dawn. He proceeded to try and pick a fight after he broke the phone on the wall, so I listened when Janice told me to move him out of the house and lock the door. He proceeded to break the window on the door and I called the police. He went next door, woke up our neighbors and tried to convince them to give him a ride to Cindy's house- to no avail. By the time he got back to the house the police were there. I assumed they would take him in for breaking our phone and window- boy was I wrong! They first argued that what he did was NOT necessarily destruction of property since he lived there he could be damaging his own property (???). They talked to him for a while and tried to placate him by driving him over to Cindy's to show him that she was ok (I was trying to follow this logic). I didn't know what drugs he had gotten into but he got into a lot of them.

Over at Cindy's house, Billy walked right past Cindy's house without even knocking on the door and made a beeline to the liquor store. He was turned away and then tried to drown himself at a nearby pond by catching his shirt on a submerged car. After the police saw all of this, incredibly they just put him back in the police car, took him BACK to our house and dumped him off in our front lawn and left!

I was dumbfounded – and mad! He just tried to drown himself and they just brought him back to our house and left US with the problem! I called the police back who told me they had no good reason to bring him in- I told them he was NOT staying at our house in that condition. The police said they had just changed shifts and had gotten no briefing on what he had done during the previous shift (???). The police suggested I go the magistrate's office to get him to issue a TDO. After the magistrate listened to what happened and I gave him a

BILLY

sworn statement, the magistrate issued the TDO and sent an officer to pick Billy up.

I was greeted with "What did you do that for?" when I got home to a tearful wife. It would be the first of many times we were torn on what to do when Billy became out of control. I told her Billy crossed the line when he broke windows and tried to drown himself- I was NOT waiting until he tried that again. Besides, they were going to take him to a hospital and evaluate him and he would be in a SAFE place while he came down from whatever he was on.

We had Sunday to regroup then we were in court on Monday for a TDO hearing. We found out Billy had a right to free attorney who, to our dismay, was arguing to have him just released! We had no attorney. We brought pictures of the damage done to windows and the phone, and relayed the jumping in the pond debacle. Billy's attorney argued that since we had planned to replace the windows, Billy's breaking of the windows caused "no real harm". He argued that the phone could be repaired and the story about the pond was hearsay (Billy was NOW denying he intended to kill himself).

The group of psychiatrists, community service workers and the Loudoun County Judge took a ton of time to explain rules and procedures but only a moment to find that Billy did not meet the criteria to be TDOed- and he was free to go. It was obvious he was having cravings again, and he immediately ran out in front of traffic in front of Route 15 and was nearly hit by a car.

Soon after that we took him to Dr. V. who took one look at him and refused to give him any Adderall. It was clear he had been abusing it for a long time, and he was not going to prescribe any more while he was in this condition. He came home then immediately left for the shopping center. His friend Mateo's dad was there and to ease the tension at home agreed to take Billy to his house for the night.

Tuesday afternoon rolled around and Billy called Janice for a ride home. The peace was short-lived – as soon as he got home he immediately started tearing up the house looking for Adderall. Janice called me to come home immediately so I took off from work after I called the police to meet us at the house.

I got home to a madhouse. Billy was ranting and roaming through a house that looks like a twister hit it. The police were trying to calm him down and talking about criteria. "Just take him" I told them- but it was not that easy. Billy had to show that he was an immediate threat to himself or others to be TDOed, and what he had done to that point did not meet criteria. Also, in keeping with the criteria, his TDO charge on Monday had NO BEARING on this event.

Fortunately, the officer there was sympathetic to us and looked for evidence that he would meet this criterion. As he passed the upstairs bathroom, he saw REDRUM scrawled on the bathroom mirror. This was MURDER spelled backwards. The officer felt that, in his opinion, this met the TDO criteria. I saw that there was a great deal of discretion when interpreting that criterion, but I was not arguing and was grateful. They cuffed him and took him out to the police car with him screaming the entire time.

As they were putting him in the squad car, they bumped his head on the car roof before they closed the door. Billy then proceeded to kick out both police car windows in the back seat with his boots, spraying the officers with

BILLY

pieces of window glass. I could not believe things escalated to this point so fast. He was charged with 3 felonies, assault on 2 officers (the flying glass I guess) and destruction of THEIR windows. Before he went to jail, they whisked him away to Poplar Springs mental hospital in Petersburg for a multiday stay- no TDO hearing for this one.

Chapter 8

Wow. If we were fooling ourselves that what we had just witnessed was a passing phase, we ceased to believe that anymore. It was almost surreal watching Billy's feet go through the police windows. There was shock and tears. Part of me was very sad it had to come to this, another part of me was relieved that he was going to be confined until they could find out what was wrong with him- we would not have to debate criteria tonight.

Billy was obviously very sick. Bipolar, schizophrenia all wrapped around a serious addiction to Adderall and DXM products. I was frustrated that Billy was charged with a felony for acting out his mental illness. If he were in a mental institution and did this he certainly would not be charged with a felony, but alas this was not the case. And why did we need him to be charged with a felony before we could get him help for his mental illness anyway?

Honestly, at that time my concern was getting to the bottom of his mental illness and addiction not the felony charge. My hope was that the felony charge would force Billy to get help he had resisted for so long. Opting out of getting help would put him in a jail cell.

We went to visit him in Poplar Springs Hospital on Father's day 2002 and he hugged us like he was never going to see us again. He said "Hell of a father's day present huh pop?" I told him I was just glad he was alive... that was a good start! There was a TDO hearing scheduled and as screwy as the first hearing was, I wondered if they were again going to let him go after a couple days claiming that he no longer "met criteria" at

BILLY

that moment. My mother encouraged us to hire a private lawyer to represent our interests so I did. The onsite judge ruled that Billy was to stay up to 13 days while he was evaluated.

I was just learning about the "criteria" in Virginia. In order to qualify for a TDO, the patient had to be an "immediate threat to himself and others", and the patient had to be released once that immediate threat had past. This new philosophy was born from a nationwide movement to give patients with mental illness the "rights" they deserved. While this law certainly prevented some persons with mental illness from being banished to mental hospitals for long periods of time at the behest of their family, it crippled the rest of us who had family members with CHRONIC mental illness. Everything regarding the new laws seemed to revolve around providing TEMPORARY relief, so if you had a LONG term continuous condition, it was like putting a band aid on a deep 12 inch gash. Ultimately, the criteria was fashioned around the rapidly decreasing state and local budget being provided for mental health- construct stricter criteria for detaining individuals and ultimately there will be fewer patients to detain and spend money on. That is the way it looked to me anyway. Protecting the "rights" of mental health patients provided the perfect excuse to provide fewer services, and dump the real problem patients in the penal system. As we saw, it did nothing to actually address an ever increasing societal problem.

Janice and I had booked a timeshare for that week, so we had to take it. Janice contracted a bad cold, and our son was confined to a mental hospital so it was not the most blissful vacation we ever had. We got to visit Billy twice a week, and the drive from the Charlottesville area to Petersburg was long one. His girlfriend Cindy had sent him encouraging emails, which since we did not have access to a printer we hand copied so Billy could read them.

While Billy was at Poplar Springs, he was placed in the under 18 section of the hospital. He was 18 at that point, but their adult section was full so that is where he wound up. His main gripe with that section was that he was not allowed to smoke. To us that seemed inconsequential, but to him it was a big deal. A few days after the hearing, Billy decided he was going to try to break out of the juvenile section and had to be restrained by member of the staff, and Billy's head was cut. He was sent to a Petersburg hospital for 9 hours before they were able to get him worked on. After all that, he remained in the juvenile section.

After the vacation, I felt free to go to Melbourne, FL on business since the judge had ordered him to stay at Poplar Springs up to 13 days. The key phrase to that order... up to 13 days. I had naively assumed the treating doctor would be consulting with us on what he felt was wrong with Billy and give us a plan of attack. After all, that is why he was in the hospital right?

I could not have been more wrong. While I was in Melbourne, FL, on day 6 of his TDO, the doctor just decided to release him on June 20. I was realizing since Billy was over the age of 18, the doctors had no real obligation to tell us anything. Frequently, they didn't. He decided Billy didn't need to be there anymore, released him and called Loudoun County Sheriff's office to drive all the way to Petersburg, VA, pick him up and take him to jail.

Now in Loudoun County facing a felony charge, we felt we had to get a lawyer and defend him. We knew that if

BILLY

he was found guilty of a felony as an adult it could have far reaching effects on the rest of his life. We got a lawyer "team" who was new to Leesburg to see if we could get him out and into treatment. Within a few days, we found the jail would not give him his medication. The lawyer team informed us they could set a court hearing and, for just $350, see if they could get an order for them to give him his prescription medication. It was a good amount of money, they told me, but it will be worth it when he gets his proper medication (????). We declined this offer. I was now realizing how easy it would be to become emotionally and financially bankrupt unless we set limits on what we COULD do and what we needed to do. Billy was released June 26 so the issue was mute. Hearings awaited.

Chapter 9

We bonded Billy out of jail so we could get him into a rehab program. Before we got him home, I called Kaiser and BEGGED them to provide someone who could see Billy.

I remember choosing Kaiser Permanente as our health care provider because in 2001 our family had been relatively medication and hospital free. I had no idea that they would not cover rehab expenses at all, nor did I care about that when I made the decision in May 2002. Now because I chose Kaiser at that time, I was stuck with them for a year. They finally agreed to have a clinician talk with him, but it turned out to be a bad experience. The clinician kept touching Billy in an uncomfortable way until Billy refused to talk to him anymore.

By the weekend the Robotussin withdrawals had kicked into full gear. Janice left to go to work, and Billy conned me into getting Delsym for him (he said it was a safe substitute for Robotussin- boy was I fooled). By noon he started rolling on the floor and talking in deep Satanic tones. I called for Janice to come home and we were both wrestling with him before long. He was claiming that he was Leviathan and doing the devil's work.

We finally calmed him down and started watching a DVD together when he suddenly declared he wanted to go see a movie with his girlfriend Cindy. She wanted to see Lilo and Stich and he wanted to go now and have US give him cash enough to pay for tickets and snacks. I told him there was NO WAY I was going to do that when he was in throes of addiction- he would go straight to the pharmacy and get Robotussin with the money!

BILLY

He went downstairs and called Cindy and told her they were going to a movie – I told him that wasn't going to happen. He told her he had to hang up because he was going to fight his father.

We had an incredible battle. He attacked me and I got him in a body hold and it took all my strength to hold him. While I had him in an arm lock, Janice grabbed the ties and tied his feet, and then I was able to tie his arms. I urged Janice to call the police, but she did not want him to go back to jail even before we got a chance to get him in rehab. We managed to give him a sedative and we were able to get some sleep that night.

The next morning Billy woke up at 11 am, and I decided to call a mutual friend of ours who was Billy's age named Jayson. Jayson worked at the thrift store with Janice and was a good guy, and Billy seemed to like him. Billy asked to go to a movie with Jayson in the afternoon, and since he was going with Jayson we let him go. Before they got out of the neighborhood however, Billy demanded that Jayson take him to the drug store to get him Robotussin. When Jayson said no way, Billy leapt out of the car with money in hand and started jogging to the store alone.

Jayson came racing back to the house to let us know what happened. We dropped what we were doing and headed to Countryside shopping center. By the time we got there he had already hitched a ride to the pharmacy and bought and ingested enough Robotussin to swim in. We had to do something- but what? As far as I was concerned, mixing Adderall and Robotussin of great quantities can be lethal, and Billy knows this so this is really at threat to himself. As we saw already, Loudoun County Mental Health and the Loudoun police didn't see it that way. If we called the police they would tell us he didn't meet criteria to be TDOed, or did he meet the criteria to be arrested. We would have to wait until he was having convulsions before we could get them to believe he met medical criteria. They did admit that if he became unconscious he would have then indeed have met criteria.

We decided to tie him up and take him to Behavioral Health Services Hospital in Richmond. They told us that if we brought him in and told them about his crazy, addictive behavior that they would take him in. If we could tie him up with ties, we could drive him the 2 and a half hours and get him checked in before the convulsions start. As we were closing in on him in the shopping center, we got some surprise help from a couple who volunteered to help us tie him up so we could get him some help. I would bet they had run into a similar predicament themselves at one time. So with me, my wife, Jayson and this helpful couple that happened to be driving by, we were able to hold him down so we could tie him up. During the scuffle someone called the police and again I knew we would have to give them our best argument if we were to have a chance at TDOing him.

The police starting by telling me I had no right to restrain Billy, I was denying him his freedom and that was a crime. I told the officer that I was going to save my son from dying and if that was a crime they could arrest me (I would learn the hard way that in order to get the right thing done, you had to challenge the "rule" or "criteria" sometimes). We moved him under a shady tree but he would not drink any water because it would interact with all the Robotussin and take away the "high". The female office attempted to placate him by telling Billy that the TDO decision was up to a judge and the judge may just release him, so not to be mad at her (Billy later

BILLY

took this to mean the judge WOULD release him)! Maybe that deflected some of the anger from Billy, but it sure did not help anything.

Eventually we got the officers to take Billy in for a TDO and fortunately Billy voluntarily accepted the TDO. He is taken to Inova Mount Vernon Hospital in Alexandria from 2 July to 10 July. We were surprised when the attending physician wanted to change all of Billy's medication, even though it conflicted with the medication Billy was already on. We encouraged the doctor to speak with Billy's psychiatrist, but he was not interested in doing that! As we would see many times, the attending psychiatrists at TDOs rarely were interested in what the previous psychiatrist prescribed, or what the consequences of prescribing conflicting medications would be. I felt part of the reason was because they knew they would only be stuck with the patient for no more than 3 days, so if they were going to flip out it would not be on their watch.

While there, Billy observed one young man who kept to himself who was very quiet. One night he went into his room, turned on his hard core industrial music and minutes later came out and smashed all the computers in the facility! Since he was mentally ill and in a facility, there were no legal charges against the young man. Ironic, I thought, that Billy had had a similar manic moment, but Billy was now charged with 3 felonies for breaking the windows on the Police cruisers! If Billy were properly restrained and taken to a mental hospital at the time, he would have had no charges. On the flip side, I realized, he would ALSO be released after 3 days with no incentive to get help under the current system.

As backward as the system was, WE had to figure out how to deal within its criteria if we were going to help our son. Clearly the personnel in it had no drive to change anything. For the time being, the only way to get and keep Billy on a better path was to keep jail time hanging over his head.

When Billy got out he agreed to go to a day rehabilitation program on July 11. We didn't give him a lot of choice. It started at 7:30 am and it was within the DC beltway, but that is when the program started so that is what he was going to do. The first day was rocky- we stayed at a motel next to the day program rehab program and trying to get him to stay put was a battle. We knew that if he left to go anywhere with anyone he would soon be conning them to getting alcohol for him. The first day was a struggle for him, the second day went much better but it was obvious he was struggling to remember or concentrate on anything. By the following Wednesday the instructor of the class called us to let us know that Billy was being so sarcastic he was just one step away from getting kicked out of the class. Even while I was on the phone with the counselor, Billy was being sarcastic about the program! Despite my doubts, there was no way I was going to just WITHDRAW Billy from the program – if he got kicked out he got kicked out.

BILLY

Chapter 10

On July 10th Janice took Billy back to the Kellar School and warned him that one more outburst would get him kicked out, so he really needed to get his act together or he was facing jail immediately. Janice dropped Billy off at 7:25 am, only to get a call 90 minutes later.

It was the Kellar program- Billy was again disrupted class and he was out- come get him. I took off work (again) and when we went to pick Billy up he stared into space like a zombie. He wouldn't talk to anyone, so the program director called the Arlington Police to take him to the hospital for precautionary reasons.

In Loudoun the police would have almost immediately have told us that since he was not a threat to himself or others they could not do anything. On this day in Arlington, the counselors were quickly able to talk Billy into going to the local hospital. I have to admit, I had to wonder what the hospital was going to be able to do for him.

Billy arrived at the hospital at around 10 am and placed in a room until a doctor was available. While we were waiting, he awakened from his zombie state and now was angry that he was at the hospital. He called his girlfriend Cindy repeatedly and exaggerated how badly he was being treated. As he became more agitated, he began getting loud and started to threaten to break out. When I tried to flag down a doctor or nurse to see him (and help keep order) I could not get anyone's attention. I wondered, if they are not going to TDO him, then what are we doing here desperately trying to calm Billy down? I thought- what a waste of time this is. Just following someone's suggestion blindly was not going to work in this case, as many times we were led down dead end alleys so someone ELSE would have to worry about Billy. After several hours we got a nurse to talk to Billy, and she just told Billy he needed to "straighten up because he had his whole life ahead of him". Sweet thought but nothing he had not heard a hundred times already. I told Janice we have had enough of this and we should leave to see if they might have an opening at Pathways Rehabilitation Center in Annapolis, MD. I had called them earlier and they told me they did have a bed, but it was primarily for juveniles under 18 years of age. Even though Billy was 19, they might be able to make an exception and accept him.

Again Billy told us before he could go to Annapolis he needed to go home first to get his clothes. By this time I knew better than to accommodate that request because once he got home I would not be able to drag him out into the car and go anywhere. So at 4 pm we got on the road to Annapolis and got a room there after we set up an appointment for the next morning.

We got Billy to the appointment and fortunately it went well and the Pathways counselor told us she thought Pathways could do Billy some good. He started the 10 - 30 day program that day. We were relieved and hopeful and left him there on July 11 and returned home to Sterling for a restful night's sleep.

We came back on Saturday to participate in the family time there. Billy was doing OK, but still seemed a little standoffish. We figured- he can fake it until he makes it. After all, where he was at was the best place for him- better than jail and certainly better than being home where he could sneak off and feed his Robotussin and alcohol addictions.

BILLY

Our relief that Billy was in a rehab center was shortlived. On Sunday night, we got a call from a manic Billy who had drunk way too much coffee at an Alcoholics Anonymous meeting and had run off from the meeting. He was now in an undisclosed building talking crazy. Aliens were now guiding his thoughts and he was thinking of joining them. Life was not worth living here, he said.

We noted the number on the caller ID and immediately called the Annapolis police. We traced down the number with their help and pleaded with them to get him before he hurt himself. We managed to stay on the phone with him long enough to have them apprehend him before he acted on any of his threats.

In the state of Maryland, there were not Temporary Detention Orders as they were defined to be in Virginia. The police there did not even consider taking him in for the threats. Instead the returned him to Pathways who declared that since Billy had been away from the premises for more than an hour he was now kicked out of the program. Billy refused to go back into the facility, and he was sleeping on Pathways lawn when we came to pick him up at midnight that night. All I could think at that point was- now what? We get him into a rehab facility, he acts up and gets himself kicked out, and now thinks he can lounge around the house while he schemes to feed his Robotussin and alcohol addiction. I didn't want him to go back to jail, but I felt very frustrated and was running out of options.

I was now wondering if postponing Billy's felony hearing was such a good idea. All it was doing was just giving Billy more time to feed his addictions, get in more trouble and create more headaches for us. Counselors were not offering any real solutions ("Billy's recovery is up to Billy"). The mental health community could not agree on what mental illness he had. By this time, several psychiatrists said he WAS bipolar, several others said not. Worse, there was still no test to resolve the issue. It was suggested that if we could get Billy totally clean of the drugs and the alcohol that they would be able to make a better diagnosis. It reminded me of step one of a Chilton's auto repair book that said "Remove engine".

When Billy got home, he again started to go downhill. On August 4, after an Sunday night AA meeting, Billy was planning on going to a movie with his girlfriend Cindy. When we picked him up, he seemed extremely edgy and agitated. He started to demand cash and stated that he really didn't care whether he went to a movie with his girlfriend or not. That was a big red flag. Skeptical, I told him the only way he was going to the movies was if I bought his movie ticket by credit card and he was getting no cash. After we picked up Cindy, he then changed the plan to now go to Starbucks. Cindy was visibly upset with this plan as she wanted to go to the movies. We gave him $3 cash and dropped them off at the Starbucks.

Suspicious, I drove the car up to the Giant and staked it out. Amazingly, we saw him charging up from the Starbucks straight for the Giant to buy Robotussin. I intercepted him, but by this time he told me he was going to buy it and I couldn't stop him. He walked in and out of the video store, and Cindy intercepted him and begged him to stop and not get any Robotussin. He told her that getting Robotussin meant more to him now than anything and he was going to get it. He went in the store and I tailed him, and when he tried to buy it I begged the lady at the register not to sell it to him and she pulled it. He grabbed the bottle and a scuffle

BILLY

ensued and the police were called. Billy walked out of the Giant empty handed and then sat on the bench outside of the store, like we were going to forget what just happened and then he could try again. The police showed up and thankfully it was the SAME officer who TDOed him in June, so he TDOed him on the spot even though he had not drank a drop of Robotussin.

How fortunate was that. We got to TDO him WITHOUT worrying if he was going to die on an overdose. As much as I wish that this could happen every time, I knew that the officer had to stretch his boundaries to do the right thing. Billy voluntarily agreed to the TDO and was committed to Inova Mount Vernon Hospital for 9 days.

By this time we recognized that the addiction and mental illness were chronic problems that were going to take a long time to battle. Billy did well for a while, but on Sunday night September 16, Billy again asked to see a movie with his girlfriend Cindy. Billy was still talking about how "cool" it was to watch a movie on Robo because the movie became three dimensional to him then. Throwing out any embarrassment, I had previously went around to the stores where Billy had bought/stolen Robotussin and alcohol and asked that they PLEASE call us if Billy is seen trying to buy Robotussin products as these things will kill him! Sunday night we got a call from the Countryside CVS that Billy had bought Robotussin at their stores and said he was headed to the movies. We called the Police and fortunately they were very cooperative with us and surrounded the theater he was in. Unfortunately, they told us that unless Billy ADMITTED to abusing Robotussin they could not take him in and TDO him. There was no test for Robotussin consumption at that time. Again, I told the officers of the call I got from CVS and the fact that if Billy mixed Robotussin with his prescription Adderal it could be deadly- meeting the criteria of a threat to self. They pulled Billy and Cindy from the movies and questioned him. He had that characteristic eye twitch and squint that we immediately recognized when he was using. After a 20 minute talk with Janice, he admitted to taking the Robotussin and was TDOed.

On one hand I felt bad for his girlfriend Cindy being in the middle of all this craziness. On the other hand she seemed to be tolerating all of this drug and alcohol abuse without telling us anything quite well. We felt that if she truly loved Billy- and she had to stick by him through all this- she needed to step up and try to actually HELP him instead of looking the other way when he started using. We knew though this was a lot to ask of a 19 year old girl. This too was about to change.

BILLY

Chapter 11

While we were going through the daily battles, I decided I needed to learn more about bipolar disorder and try to understand why his addictions were all consuming. I signed up for NAMI's Family to Family classes that lasted 12 weeks. I sure learned a lot, and learned that there were a lot of families who went through this battle. A great class- I would recommend it anyone. It was easy to get totally absorbed in the day-to-day crises and NEVER make any progress on the big picture- like getting him to STAY at a stable point.

Tuesday night October 8th started out like just another night. Billy and Anthony were going to the bookstore to get a few books together. Around 8 pm he called from the bookstore and asked if I would buy him a book on witches- I said no. He and Anthony were supposed to call when they were ready to come home.

The story on Anthony was that he had successfully completed rehab and was interested in drawing his own comics. He had injured his leg and had trouble walking, but we agreed to let him stay with us if he could act as a mentor for Billy. We had yet to realize that ex-addicts had relapses, sometimes frequently, and ask anyone around them to aid them in hiding it.

We got a call at about 8:30 pm from Billy's girlfriend Cindy that he had just called her from Wal-mart. Billy had found out that his girlfriend was pregnant and he promised her that he would quit the drugs and the DXM so he could keep it together enough to support the baby. He had failed. He was throwing up and said he was going to kill himself for sure this time. He had taken bottles of Robotussin and alcohol and was going off to die. We immediately got a call after that from Anthony that Billy had run off and left him. We jumped into action and raced to pick up Anthony near the bookstore and then to Walmart. On the way we called the police to see if we could track him down.

We got there minutes later and talked with the Wal-mart manager who saw Billy make a call from the pay phone then run off the large hill across the parking lot- a hill we dubbed "Robotussin Hill". Based on Billy's history, the local police called in dogs and a helicopter to look for him. Unlike previous episodes, time was of the essence because he took a lethal dose of Robotussin and alcohol, and of course it was mixed with his MOA (Adderall).

The police started a search with the dogs and asked that we just wait in the parking lot (else we might throw off the dogs). I told them my son might be dying right now and I was not going to be standing in a parking lot while that was happening. I looked at the back lot of Lowes first, under sheds and trailers, and then made my way up to the top of the hill where I spotted a marshy pond at the bottom of the hill.

I can't tell you I scared I was that my son may actually be in there. He was just 19 and way too young to die. I prayed to God harder than I ever prayed that we would find him in time to save him.

I noticed a car had stopped at an adjacent road in an attempt to help a deer that had been hit. I also noticed there were thick woods across that road and I hoped Billy had not made it there yet, else the police would never find him in time. I made my way to the car and asked the driver if he had seen a 19 year old who was

BILLY

5'11" 140 lbs and he said "Does he look like the guy right behind you?"

It was Billy. He was wobbling and seemed very confused, but he WAS walking. He walked over to the downed deer while I desperately tried to wave down someone with a cell phone to get the police over before he bolted into the thick woods. Imagine that- with the local police scouring the area with dogs and helicopters, I was the one who found him- and NOT by sitting in a parking lot!

The police showed up minutes later and rushed him to the hospital. They pumped his stomach and amazingly he made it through without any damage. He was extremely fortunate.

The next day we were again before a judge petitioning that Billy be TDOed. I thought- what if I could not take off work AGAIN – would that mean there was no petitioner and therefore they would just let him go? Anyway, Billy looked like he had just been through a war. His girlfriend Cindy took her time to come to the hearing with us, which Billy did not fight. She asked the judge- why do you keep giving out a TEMPORARY detention order over and over when he obviously needs long term help. Why can't you order him to the hospital for a month?

Cindy said what all of us had wondered since June. Obviously Billy had demonstrated over the last 5 months that he had a chronic addiction to DXM and alcohol, yet the only thing that could be done for him was to give him a 3 day Temporary Detention Order over and over. What was worse was that everyone in the system seemed to have accepted that this was "the way it was", even the court appointed attorney had to acknowledge that he was just "doing his job" by trying to get Billy out of the TDO, even though it was obvious that that was the worst thing for him.

Billy was dispatched to the Inova Fairfax Hospital in Falls Church. He was then discharged 6 days later for failure to participate in activities. He went back to Loudoun County jail for failure to honor his capius of not using drugs; they kept him there until 31 October. Unfortunately, Cindy lost the baby during that time due to natural causes. A part of us was relieved because neither one of them was in anyway prepared to take care of a baby. We also felt that if she had the baby WE would have eventually been asked to raise it.

After discussing matters with the Court, we arranged for him to get of jail to attend the Serenity House in Fredericksburg, VA. A week earlier a Serenity House representative interviewed him in jail and agreed to accept him. Since we had an HMO, there was no insurance coverage of this rehabilitation facility. We drove him down first thing on 1 November and even though he had some apprehension he went.

Two days later we went down for a Saturday family visit, and we brought his girlfriend down with us. We were surprised when we got to drive him to the mall for lunch, and the visit went well. After we left, Cindy mentioned that she thought she saw seeds in Billy's mouth, we hoped she was mistaken.

No sooner that we got back to Sterling we got a call from Serenity House. Billy had refused to cooperate with the staff and now he was completely out of his head. They later traced it down to him ingesting Datura weed from the next door lot. Incredibly, they asked me

BILLY

to come down to Fredericksburg and pick him up at his maniacal worst and bring him back home.

I told them there was NO WAY I was going to do that! The program director then told me she knew the right words to say to get him into the hospital, I said I hoped so because someone who is out of his head and violent has no business being out in the street!

He was taken to Mary Washington hospital in Fredericksburg where he was latched down to the bed. He had a full time babysitter there to make sure he didn't hurt himself. His older brother Eric went to visit him and reported that he didn't know who anyone was for days.

He was then transferred to Snowden Mental Health Facility around the corner after he became aware of who he was again. After initially promising to try to get Billy into Western State Hospital for long term care, they later surprised us by quickly releasing him with no explanation and no chance to discuss ANY follow up care. They basically gave him his belongings and pushed him out the door, locking the other side before they had to talk to us at all.

Chapter 12

November 13, 2002 was just another in a long string of disappointments. We had a son who had a bad mental and addictive disorder and all the "center" he ended up did was push him out the door without giving us a clue where we go from there. We got him out of jail to go to a rehabilitation center, he took datura while he was there, went out of his mind and NOW he was simply DISCHARGED from Snowden. Here he is- we don't want to deal with him, good luck with him, <click>.

Was he cured? No way. Did he have a plan to get better? Nope. Janice and I wondered- what do we do now? Although the BEST place for Billy to be was long term hospitalization where he would not be able to abuse substances, we knew we were not going to get that. We heard a quiet ticking in our head- how long do we have to do something with him before he starts stealing DXM and alcohol again?

Added to that was our constant dialog with the insurance company. How many days were they going to authorize? Were they going to surprise us by not paying their portion and forcing us to appeal? Were they going to complain that we didn't call them first before TDOing him (as if we had ANY time to do that...)?

What else could we do except try to get him in another rehab center. We told the court that we were going to do that to get him released, so all we could do was try again. With Anthony's help, we contacted the Phoenix House in Washington DC and through the help of Loudoun Mental Health we arranged for Billy to report there on December 9. Amazingly, we got Loudoun

BILLY

County Mental Health to agree to pay for it. All we had to do is keep Billy calm until then – again if he refused to go to treatment he would go back to jail.

I took the pre-emptive measure of going to court to ask the judge to amend his order to include OTHER rehab centers, such as Phoenix house. He did that and wished Billy the best.

The next day the OTHER judge who issued the original order got the information that Billy was released from Serenity House (a few weeks too late to say the least....). Apparently he did not speak with the judge who just amended the order, as the original judge issued a capius for Billy for failing to honor the original order. The next day police showed up at the house to take him to jail. I was furious- we were planning to take him to rehab in a few days!! Ultimately, I bonded Billy out until he could make it to rehab. I was realizing that when the County made a mistake and it did not negatively affect THEM, nothing was going to be done unless WE pitched a fit about it. I also realized that the communication between residing judges was something less than perfect.

We were advised by LCMH to DROP Billy's insurance so he would be eligible for county sponsored rehab programs. They told us that is why they were not able to help him before. When we did that, he was accepted at the Phoenix House.

All was on track until the night of December 6 that is. Cindy had come over to visit but asked me to take her home by 10 pm because she had to go to class the next morning. It was a work night so I also wanted to take her home before it got too late.

Billy asked if he could talk with her another 15 minutes- I said fine but then it was time to take her home. He was mad she wanted to go home, but I told him he needed to respect her wishes and that was that. I took Cindy home, and then came back to a son who sliced his face into pieces with a razor blade! Initially I was upset that neither Janice nor Anthony noticed this, but I realized if he did this silently in his room, how would anyone upstairs know? Before we could call the ambulance Billy agreed to have us take him to Loudoun Hospital. He wanted the cell phone to call Cindy and tell her it was HER fault he did this...I took the phone from him. Fortunately Billy agreed to voluntarily TDO at Northern Virginia Community Hospital off of Gallows Road.

Then we learned that this TDO, according to Anthony who had been there, was going to cause the Phoenix House to reconsider accepting Billy on 9 December. NVCH let the Phoenix House know Billy was in the hospital for self mutilation. We tried to call them, but they would not talk to us and would only offer to send us a pamphlet. We needed to know if they were going to reconsider the circumstances and let Billy enter the program. We finally heard back that they would reconsider, but now they would not talk to us. I desperately tried working with them through Loudoun County Mental Health, but no one would ever return my calls. I really did lose it on the last day for reconsideration the lone LCMH worker who could do something was at an all day "off site" and no one could take the call.

So much for reconsideration- I could not even TALK with the staff! Now we had to look elsewhere and hope the court did not find Billy for failure to comply with a court order. We called the Serenity House in Fredericksburg and fortunately they agreed to take him

BILLY

back. Given the history that we had just experienced, I thought I should find a backup just in case we ran into any more "surprises".

That was a smart thing to do. On the day Janice drove to Fredericksburg, the director of the Serenity House announced at the 11th hour that she didn't take "dual diagnosis" patients (those that have an addiction AND another disorder) and refused to let Billy into the program. She knew Billy's history for 45 days and NOW she decided to invoke her "dual diagnosis" rule. What great timing!

By this point I was getting better about coming up with a plan "B" for rehab plans. I had taken the liberty of calling another rehabilitation center in Winchester, VA called Edgehill and fortunately they had one bed left. They did not take insurance so we would have to pay our own money upfront, but at that point we were out of options. I caught up with Janice and Billy that night in Fredericksburg and we decided to spend the night and change course and head to Winchester. After a rough night where all Billy did was try to sneak out of the room and buy cough syrup, we made it to Edgehill on 15 December.

Edgehill accepted Billy that day and again we were cautiously hopeful. By the time we came to visit him on Saturday, we were told he already had a "house rest" on Friday for taking Robotussin from a pharmacy while they were walking to the nightly AA meeting! I thought- he has to pass a drug store with Robotussin and Corocidin on open shelves every night to get to the AA meeting? Sounded like a recipe for disaster to me.

I brought Anthony and one of Billy's old girlfriends (Beth) with me for the Saturday visit, and later Billy admitted that what he wanted to do was take someone hostage so he could get a big supply of Robotussin and alcohol. By Christmas Eve, less than a week later, we got a call from the director, that they felt Billy was not a good "match" for the program and were releasing him. We got this letter from the director:

William Hawthorne voluntarily [entered] EdgeHill on December 15, 2002. After several days in residence, several of Mr. Hawthorne's peers came to staff to advise [that] he was drinking cough syrup by the bottles at the local convenience store. Mr. Hawthorne admitted it was true [and] that he did not think he could function without [DXM].

As you know there is not a urine screen (non-lab) test for [DXM]. In addition to his addiction we felt he needed more that what EdgeHill could offer him. We are not a medical model and it is staff's opinion that Mr. Hawthorne needs mental health assistance as well as substance abuse education and living skills.

He was not terminated from EdgeHill for non-compliance. He was very cooperative and honest. It is our hope that Mr. Hawthorne gets the medical attention he needs so he will be able to focus on his 12 step recovery program.

And – how on earth were we to do that? The most we could get out of a mental hospital was a 3 day TDO from psychiatrists who constantly contradicted each other in their diagnosis and medications then suddenly released him when they were tired of dealing with him. And .. they told us they could deal with his mental illness but not his addictions!! Expecting us to somehow "find" the perfect institution that would deal with his addiction as well as his mental illness was proving almost

BILLY

impossible. We were starting to feel like this was worse than if Billy had an incurable, terminal disease.

When we picked Billy up, he was not in good shape, and he actually told me he felt like dying. We called LCMH in hopes that we could possibly get him TDOed so he would not attempt to kill himself again, but we were told that the "threat" was probably too dated- by the time we got him back to Leesburg from Winchester it would be more than an hour and thus he would not meet criteria. He would need to repeat his threat again when he got to Leesburg to be eligible for a TDO. Exasperated, we just told them forget it we will bring him home and if he does hurt himself we will call (and not a moment before). That brought 2002 to an end and we felt like we had been through a lifetime of battles already!

Chapter 13

Well we had just been through hell and it had only been 7 months since Billy went off the deep end. The only good thing about 2003 was that we could now get Billy back ON our insurance (and it was NOT an HMO) so he could get his medication and he would not get $5000 bills from mental hospitals anymore. The new insurance now paid for trips to rehabilitation facilities along with his meds and doctor visits. Dropping his insurance was the dumbest advice we ever got.

We had run out of rehabilitation houses to try for the moment. We called insurance and got a new psychiatrist who worked out of Reston. However, as we moved into early January 2003 Billy seemed to be slinking back to his old bad habits. Now he was depressed and in a bad mood all the time, he refused to do any school work or get a job. His face was gaunt and again he was staying up all night and sleeping all day. I caught him riding up to the CVS at 5:30 pm in 20 degree weather, then swearing he just wanted to "get some exercise". By the end of the month it was obvious he was getting drugs somehow, then we found a huge stash of empty Robotussin bottles in the hamper in his bathroom that proved it. With no money, it was obvious he had stolen them.

Meanwhile, I had been trying to work with his new psychiatrist to get him into an insurance approved rehabilitation center. He told me not to RUSH and put him somewhere where he would be kicked out quickly again. I countered that he was sliding downhill rapidly and we needed to act quickly before he got stuck in the endless TDO cycle again or even worse succeeded in

BILLY

killing himself! I begged him to move faster but my pleas fell on deaf ears.

On Saturday January 25th Billy asked me to take him to Cindy's house. After the last TDO she obviously was growing tired of the continuous trips to the hospital and Billy's addictive behavior had cooled the relationship. Who could blame her? So I didn't really trust that Billy was invited over. I told Anthony to call Cindy and warn her that Billy was coming over. Over the month of January he had gotten progressively meaner and I was not going to tolerate him threatening her or pressuring her to see him.

Sure enough, when we got to Cindy's apartment I could tell there would be problems. Billy wanted me to drop him off and keep driving... I was not about to do that. I dropped him off and her mother immediately waved for me to come back. Cindy told him he could not come in and it was over between them. Billy asked why not and it was on. She closed the glass door and Billy took a rock and sent it right through the door. He tried to throw a rock at the second floor window, but I blocked his throw. I yelled at him to stop, then he bolted for my car (which was still running) and unfortunately the keys were still in it. He tried to put it in gear but I fought him until he agreed to get out of the car. I locked the car and chased him out of the back of the apartments and onto a path. He apparently was trying to get back to the Good Shepherd Thrift Store where Janice was working where in his mind he could hide out from the police.

Running, I followed him and periodically he would stop and threaten to stab me if I got closer. I told him I was not going to push him to do anything but I also was not leaving. We passed a couple going through the tunnel and I yelled for them to please call the police quickly.

He made it to a culvert pipe where he tried to fit himself through the bars in his thick trench coat and run through the pipe and make a getaway, but he was too big to do that. We made it to a hill where I finally talked him into putting the knife away and he started crying. He blamed himself for Cindy losing the baby, and he was so sorry he had become so addicted to DXM and alcohol. I finally was able to hug him and walk with him to a nearby street. Within 5 minutes the police converged on us and took him off to the Loudoun County mental hospital for yet another hearing. I was just glad he got there alive this time.

Billy was voluntarily admitted to NVMH, and after 3 days the doctors tricked him into coming into a room so the police could take him to jail. Billy was actually charged with assault by Cindy's mother, who was inside the apartment during the entire incident. She quickly dropped the charge when Billy's lawyer proposed compensating her $400 for the broken door. Little did we know that dropped charge would come back to haunt him later. Needless to say, it was OVER between Billy and Cindy.

Once he got back to jail, we asked ourselves- maybe this IS the best place for him. After all, if he can't stay in a rehab for more than a few days, this would be better than releasing him and allowing him to sneak out of the house and get more DXM/alcohol. The balance breaker for us though was realizing he would get NO mental health care in jail, and in fact his bipolar behavior would probably be exacerbated in jail. After all, he would just serve his time and with no other help he would almost certainly go right back to his addictions. We decided to work with Billy's attorney to get Billy into a long term rehabilitation program.

BILLY

Billy stayed in the Loudoun County jail for a month, and frankly, I think at that point he needed to. He was getting himself kicked out of all the rehabs we had sent him to, but he could NOT get himself kicked out of jail. He learned he could not talk back to people and he would be FORCED to detox himself from the DXM and the alcohol. After a few weeks, he was desperate enough to agree to go to a 60 day program. We arranged for him to meet with a representative from Deep Run Lodge of Goldvein, VA, just south of Manassas. We wanted to have them keep him for 90 days but our insurance would only cover 60 days/year- so 60 days it was. The Circuit court judge released him to attend Deep Run lodge for 60 days on Feb 25, 2003.

Getting him down to Goldvein did not go smoothly. We stopped in Manassas to get him a lip pin, but when we got to Deep Run he told us he didn't want to go. We told him if that was the way he felt we would leave him for the police to pick him up and he could stay in jail for months. He turned around and went back in. He told us another inmate (who was also bipolar) told him he HAD to take this opportunity or he might not make it out- Billy listened. That inmate ended up committing suicide 5 days later.

Then the counselor asked him if he had abused any drugs over the last 30 days and surprisingly he said yes! Apparently an inmate had snuck in prescription drugs and of course Billy had to trade for that. That is the LAST place we expected him to get drugs. We were beginning to believe if he were on the moon he would find drugs somehow.

Chapter 14

Billy entered Deep Run knowing that if he were kicked out he would go straight back to jail. Also, he was out in the middle of nowhere so he could not take a side trip to the pharmacy. Janice and I got to visit every Saturday, but since Janice had to work most Saturdays, they allowed her to come and visit him on Wednesdays. He seemed to be doing ok – he had gotten to go sledding with other kids his age, play softball and basketball and hopefully learn a thing or two.

The center had tutors for those who were missing school, but Billy was doing online school with Alpha Omega. I brought all the lessons down to him to work on, but he worked on none of it. Things were going alright until our week 4 visit, when Billy was talking to me then decided to take off. He ran down to the creek and just sat there, and I felt I had to follow him to make sure he didn't try to kill himself. After about 45 minutes he decided to come back and made it back to the campus just in time to avoid being expelled. I thought- why did he have to do this during MY visit?

During week 6 he had to go back to court in Loudoun County. Janice picked him up on a weekday, took him to his hearing where the judge was glad to hear that Billy was still in the program. On the way back he asked to stop at a park then refused to get back in the car. After 30 minutes of pleading, Billy finally agreed to get back in the car and again just made the time deadline and again was NOT expelled!

After 60 days Billy was released. He had made it through 60 days and did not get expelled, and although he had his rough spells he did make it through. We were proud of him! He had requested to go live with his sister in Louisiana after he got out, and we all thought that was a great idea where he could help take care of his nephew Chris. After speaking with his probation officer, we seemed to get concurrence on that idea.

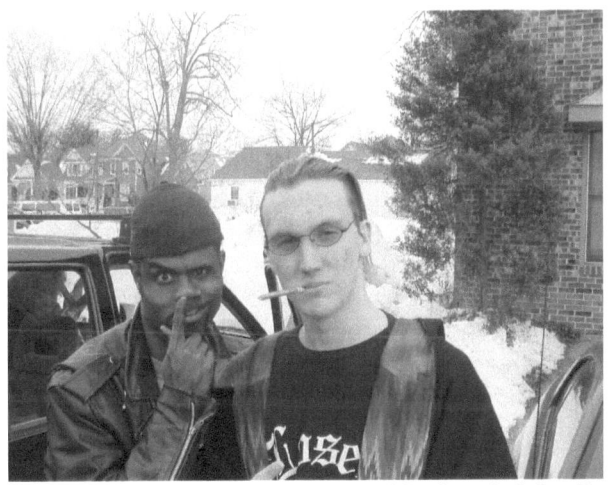

Billy and Anthony clowning around before left for Deep Run Rehabilitation in Goldvein, VA in February 2003

When Billy reported to court after he was released from rehab, it was a TOTALLY different story. Now all his probation officer wanted to do was put him back in jail! I called his probation officer and asked her what was going on, she said "Mr. Hawthorne, 90 days ago you BEGGED for him to go to jail!" I told her that was 90 days ago and he had come a long way since then and deserved to have a chance to make it after completing his 2 month rehab.

In my opinion, probation services then played dirty. After getting a fair report from Deep Run (Billy completed rehab, but didn't necessarily complete all the goals they hoped for), probation services called Deep Run and pressured them into writing a more NEGATIVE report that they could parlay into a "failure to complete" so they would not have to deal with him on probation again.

Probation representatives pointed out that Billy failed to complete a 90 day rehab program as recommended, but the judge correctly countered that our insurance limited rehab days to 60, so Billy would not be penalized by that. Billy's attorney pointed out that the new negative report was received AFTER probation services pressured Deep Run into resubmitting a new more NEGATIVE report, and he was going to make a motion to delay the hearing until he could get Deep Run representatives on the stand to question them. With that, probation agreed to strike the report entirely from evidence.

Ultimately, the judge agreed to let Billy serve his remaining time on probation at home, but he would have to be fitted with a GPS monitor. Billy reluctantly agreed, but we felt this was much better than jail. Billy's hostility continued to build when he was fitted for ankle bracelet, to the point that he wandered out of the courthouse and we had to BEG to get back into the car to go home!

We took him home and as usual I had to go back to work and try to make up my missed time. Court proceedings had taken up a LOT of work time over the last few years, I was fortunate to be able to make it up.

BILLY

After I dropped Janice, Billy and Anthony off at home, all hell broke loose. Billy was so agitated with having to wear the ankle bracelet he attacked Anthony with a knife! Janice finally had to call the police and he again was TDOed to Northern Virginia Community Hospital. After three days, they told us they were going to move him to Northern Virginia Mental Hospital on Gallows Road because it looks like they had a bed open there. While there they started giving him Neurontin, which seemed to plunge Billy into a terrible depression. The Neurontin was administered by the attending doctor and he made it clear he didn't care what medicine Billy was on before we got to HIS hospital. Our complaints about Billy becoming extremely suicidal fell on deaf ears.

The next day Janice got a call at 4:10 p.m. It was Dr. R. He told Janice that he was releasing Billy now- he was putting him in a cab either to our house or to the Washington DC homeless shelter. He told her that, in his opinion, Billy wasn't suicidal (despite his repeated threats to the contrary). Janice then pleaded with him to at least hold him so she could pick him up, he told her the office closed at 4:15 pm and she would not make it in time. Knowing how suicidal Billy was, she pleaded with him to not give him the whole bottle of Neurontin to take with him because he already threatened to take the whole bottle and end it all now. Again the doctor said he didn't think that would happen. The doctor then gave Janice a choice- either let him put Billy in a cab and dump him in our yard or he would be dumped in front of a Washington DC homeless shelter. Janice felt she had no choice but to accept option 1.

What total arrogance and irresponsibility! We prayed during that entire cab ride and fortunately Billy did not commit suicide on the way home. We immediately called the hospital and after we had Billy sign all the endless released the hospital director told us there had been a "misunderstanding" and that doctors at their hospital would not do such a thing. I assured her it had happened and we were pissed. She offered to give him an examination "on the house" I am sure to cover their ass, but we refused.

The following two weeks was hell. Upon returning home, Billy was again fitted with a tracking device and ordered to attend an AA meeting every night, 7 days a week. In the meantime, he became extremely dark and suicidal- all he talked about was killing himself. Community corrections seemed to know nothing about mental illness (a criminal is a criminal, right?), and Billy's probation officer did not even want to talk to me about his suicidal tendencies (or anything else for that matter). Every night I snuck out of the house to use the cell phone and call Loudoun County Mental Health emergency line only to be told that a) Billy didn't meet the criteria to be helped, b) I should keep the knives hidden and c) I should just stay with him and make sure he didn't hurt himself and, oh yes, cross my fingers and hope he didn't hang or stab himself. Oh- if he actually DID hang or stab himself, he would then meet criteria and be eligible for help. I thought- why couldn't she just say "I am incompetent and you should call a national suicide hotline because we have no one here qualified to help you".

Over those 2 weeks we hid all the knives and cut down the rope swing before he used it to kill himself. I had not seen my son smile or laugh in two weeks. One particular night I could just see that he was plotting of how to kill himself after we went to bed. I suggested that when we got home we have a WWF wrestling match on the trampoline when we got home. I let him plan everything right down to the intro music and the

BILLY

announcements. Even though this really was not my thing, I went along with everything. To my relief, he started smiling and laughing again! After he executed a perfect pile driver, he confided "Dad, I think this match just saved my life". Things took a better turn after that, and he thanked me for suggesting that for the next week.

We followed this up with taking Billy back to his old psychiatrist Dr. Mark Simonds who told us that it looked like Neurontin was the WORST thing Billy could take. It was serving as a depressant and driving an already suicidal person over the edge. We saw an immediate and lasting improvement once he was off the Neurontin.

This made me even more determine to try and hold the doctor from Billy's last TDO accountable. I contacted the Department of Professional Regulation and they in turn directed me to the Office of Medical Regulation. After what seemed to be endless waiting followed by a few interviews, I got a call back that the board ruled the doctor did not do anything wrong. They wouldn't tell me what was discussed, that was confidential. What evidence was considered was confidential. The reasoning they used was confidential. I asked if Billy had indeed committed suicide on that cab ride home, would anything have been done? Possibly, I was told.

What a joke of a hearing. Confidentiality overrode all sense of protecting the public. It seemed to me it was all about protecting the doctors. Now I could see why the doctor pulled this stunt. He needed another bed and he knew there would be no repercussions on doing such a crazy thing as sending a suicidal man home with an entire bottle of medication! And I was told, if he DID commit suicide, I could sue him in court for damages (that would be just a little too late ...). Otherwise, it looked to me like there was no accountability. I wondered- how many other patients did the doctor send home or to a homeless shelter in a cab?

As I mentioned earlier, despite Community Corrections best efforts to put Billy back in jail so they would not have to fool with him, the judge ruled that he be released with a GPS monitor and attend daily AA meetings. Billy was assigned a probation officer, and she promptly informed us that she would be interfacing with Billy only- she normally didn't talk with the parents of an adult. The implication here was obvious- we babied Billy and that was contributing to his bad behavior. She reasoned that if we would just leave him alone and let him handle his own affairs as an adult, things would go better and Billy would learn responsibility. Good theory I guess from someone who didn't know Billy from a hole in the wall, but obviously this does not work with someone with a mental disorder and chronic addictions.

It was also contradictory. Billy in fact depended on us for everything. Being on house arrest, Ms M. did not allow Billy to work (the GPS monitor would catch him if he did and he would be violated). Billy was completely dependent on us for everything, especially to take him to and pick him up from all mandatory AA meetings. If we had a problem with anything she was directing- tough- she was the P.O. and she was going to have things her way. Already, it almost seemed as if she delighted in irritating us- me in particular.

As May approached, I was beginning to realize what a burden taking Billy to an AA meeting EVERY day was going to be. Also, I was not at all convinced that going to these meetings was actually helping him. I thought at first, maybe he can "fake it till he makes it". When one

BILLY

of us took him to a meeting, we had to then kill an hour or so until the meeting was over, then come home. There were no nights we could just relax at home- one of us had this responsibility every night for 4 months, rain or shine. The PO suggested that we give him a bus token to take to his own meetings, totally blind to the fact that Billy would take advantage of that time by stealing DXM or alcohol.

After one meeting in May, we both picked Billy up and asked if he would like for us to stop at a fast food place for a bite to eat. Strangely, he told us he wanted to stop at a convenience store. Though skeptical, we stopped at a gas station where he got some potato chips. As we were going out, the manager pointed out that Billy needed to pay for his bottle of Scope mouthwash (with alcohol) he stuffed in his coat! Embarrassed and not wanting to hit Billy with any more charges, we paid for the mouthwash and I put it in my coat.

I should have just given it back to store. I gave it to Janice while I drove home on Algonkian Parkway and Billy didn't say a word. One mile down the road, he leapt at Janice in the back seat and grabbed the Scope and ripped it from her hands. I grabbed his arms and we fought for the Scope while I was still driving! After breaking my turn signal, I managed somehow to dump the Scope out the window with him opening his mouth trying to get a sip as it poured out. I was amazed I didn't get in an accident. I thought about calling the police but I didn't want to again hear that now that the incident was over he no longer met any kind criteria and drive off.

Amazingly, this aberration was tracked on GPS, and the next day Billy was asked to explain himself. His PO gave Billy a warning but excused him that time. I thought- maybe this tracking thing has some potential.

The next week at a Narcotics Anonymous meeting, Billy left the GPS tracker box outside the meeting building only to find that is was gone when he got out of the meeting. We searched for it for a while before we eventually went to the local police station to report it. While we were waiting, Billy got very dark and quiet, and then asked for the keys to the car so he could listen to the radio. Janice sensed something was wrong and went with him. He later confessed he wanted to start the car and run it over a cliff!!

The box was lost and it was going to take $2500 to replace. If we didn't do it, Billy would go back to jail. If hindsight were 20/20, we would have allowed that to happen. Billy didn't seem to be getting anything out of the meetings after a month, and his attitude was awful. Honestly I was considering not paying for another monitor and have him sent back to jail, but we still felt at that point he would be worse off in jail where he would get no mental health care and we would have to fight with the medical staff constantly to have him stay on his prescription meds. Ultimately, we got a new box for him to give the 120 meetings in 120 days a chance.

BILLY

Chapter 15

During this time Janice and I were encouraged to go to Al-Anon groups also while Billy was at his AA meeting on Saturday nights. Honestly, I would have to give the Al-Anon meetings a mixed review. Many times our meetings would degenerate into personal problems people were having unrelated to addiction of love ones. Janice and I cringed when a couple argued over their checkbook there, and another lady talked about sleeping with her boss to get a 5 figure salary. Like dealing with all of Billy's therapists, we realized we would have to try a few different groups until we found one that we enjoyed and really seemed to help us.

We were encouraged to let Billy be responsible for his own messes. Yet, at every turn, just doing that alone did not seem like the right thing to do. When Billy lost his box, we could have just let probation send him back to jail to serve out the rest of his term. But if we did that, he would get no treatment and most likely would come out just as addicted as he went in while learning nothing. We felt like we had to give him a chance to get better, learn how to control his urges and adjust to his medication. After all, if he leaves meetings early or leaves the house, the GPS unit is going to track this and he will be violated.

That is only true if the probation officer chooses to look at GPS tracking reports and decides on act on them. We found that his PO did neither. As the summer wore on, we again noted Billy's mood returning to the dark side. He again covered up all the windows with black curtains and blankets, stayed to himself and was getting very little school work done. Although this was a clear sign he was again using DXM, he had no way to get it we thought. If he left the house he would be violated, and we did not notice him ever trying to do that. Somehow he must be getting DXM or alcohol during the AA meetings.

I again tried to contact his PO about our concerns, only to be reminded very curtly that she didn't talk to parents of adult clients. Also, a review of GPS tracking was going to be done at HER discretion, and we did not have any input into her decision. She would talk to our attorney about Billy often, but never us. She actually suggested giving Billy bus fare to take the bus to AA meetings, but we knew he would just jump off the bus and get alcohol or DXM. We were to later find out he was leaving his meetings as soon as we dropped him off, stealing alcohol or DXM, and making it back to the meeting before one of us came to pick him up. He knew his PO had to know this (either that or she never bothered to check the GPS reports) but just did not act on it. I couldn't help but think that she was not reviewing the GPS reports just to irritate me. Billy later disclosed that some of his tests came up "dirty" for marijuana, but his PO didn't act on it (Billy also verified that she seemed to get a thrill out of irritating me...).

Billy's 120 days of meetings was finally over on September 4, 2003 and he was granted permission to come with us to Cape Cod on vacation with us. Having to take separate vacations in the summer so someone could take Billy to his daily court ordered meetings, Janice and I were thrilled to be able to go on a vacation together and NOT have to consume our every evening going to AA meetings and getting home at 10:30 pm every night. As we found out, Billy's addiction had not even waned during the 120 days- and now he was free of the GPS monitor. his PO had already ordered Billy to take a series of follow-up rehab courses when he

BILLY

returned from vacation, but left it up to us to find these classes and have our insurance pay for it. So much for enabling his independence huh?

The honeymoon of freedom was shortlived. Billy's mood was still dark, and he covered up all the windows as soon as we got to our timeshare. He turned the air conditioning to his room on cold despite the fact that the weather was quite comfortable. His game now was to refuse to go anywhere with us, and when we would go anyway and leave him alone, he would go out and steal DXM. I refused to babysit him, I told Janice if we ruined our vacation by doing that, he would just say he wanted to go for a walk or leave at night after we were asleep and we would be preventing him from doing anything.

While Billy froze in his room, Janice and I did find time to enjoy Cape Cod going to the beach, eating out and seeing the sights. Our last night at the timeshare, Billy suddenly asked if he and I could play putt putt golf. Seeing that we had not done hardly anything all vacation together, I said sure. By the time we got to the fourth hole, he was weaving so bad he almost fell down the stairs. I turned in the putters and held him up while we crossed the street. By the time we got back to the room, he was crawling on the floor with his eyes dilated. We immediately called the ambulance that had to cajole him to be taken to the hospital even though it was obvious he really needed to go. At that time he had confessed that he took 48 Coricidin tablets (a normal person would take 2 if they had a cough to relief cough and cold symptoms).

By the time he got to the Cape Cod Hospital, he had become combative. In Massachusetts he met the criteria of being committed for the night because 48 Coricidin pills was definitely a danger to him. The attending nurses finally had to inject him with something to calm him down to get him to stop yelling at them.

We visited him the next morning and found that they had given him Haldol to calm down. His tongue started swelling and his airway was closing, but Billy told the staff he was allergic to Haldol and to give him the anticonvulsive medication (Cogentin) immediately. Fortunately the staff acted quickly and gave him the antidote and reversed the effects. That was a close call!

Billy had a major setback. When he was released days later, we went to a local zoo before leaving the area, and I noticed he was hanging back to talk to the ticket taker, asking him if he could get a permanent job there! We took him aside and asked him what was going on, he told us he didn't want to go back to Virginia where he would either go to jail or another 120+ days of AA meetings! Since he was an adult, he could make the choice of not to come back with us if we were going back to Virginia and he would take whatever consequences resulted from this.

Not wanting him to freeze in Cape Cod over the winter of not knowing anyone or have any skills, we were able to contact his sister Lisa and she agreed to again let Billy stay with her and take care of her son while she worked. We were all aware that this arrangement did not work so well before, but what else were we going to do? We drove back home, but the next morning Janice and Billy got in the car and headed to New Llano, Louisiana and we all hoped for the best.

BILLY

Chapter 16

Unfortunately, when Billy arrived in Louisiana, he immediately went back to abusing alcohol. Lisa and Todd were on an Army base housing unit in New Llano, LA. Janice and Lisa tried to stop it, but while he was drinking he didn't do anything bad enough to get himself arrested. It looked like he traded his addiction to cough syrup for an addiction to alcohol. Also, he was taking care of his nephew Chris so Lisa was reluctant to get him out of the house.

Loudoun County told me that because Billy was only charged with a misdemeanor, they would not make any effort to pick him up. However, since he violated probation, there was a capius out on him and he would be picked up and taken to jail upon coming back to Virginia. At this point I was beginning to think that in jail at least he would be isolated from DXM and alcohol enough to start some kind of recovery.

It looks like in October the drugs caught up to Anthony too. He had been leaving the house once a month to see his "family" but when we called his family no one had seen him. He would come back beaten up but deny ever using any drugs (and this is the one we got to help Billy through his sobriety?). Finally in October, I gave him the cell phone so he could call me from his work, but I never got the call. He was missing for a week. Fearing the dealers would now be able to get into the house; I terminated service to the cell phone and changed the locks. When he stumbled back in a week later, I told him that was it- he was out. After some drama, he packed his stuff and let me drop him off in downtown DC (where his "family" was?). It just showed me- sometimes the people you get to help your son through addictions can be a worse addict than he is!

In early October of 2003, Janice, Lisa, Chris and Billy all went to a rodeo in New Llano, LA. Before he got there, Billy consumed almost an entire bottle of hard liquor. When he got to the rodeo, he took Chris through the stands and went on a rant of how he hated the United States and was going to burn any American Flag he found. He followed that up by giving the finger to the flag.

Fortunately, the police flagged him down just before he got his brains beat in by many God-fearing flag loving country boys. He was arrested for being drunk and disorderly and thrown into the local jail with both whites and blacks. After he reluctantly had he long hair shaved ("welcome to the south boy"), he proceeded to tell all the blacks in his cell that they should all go back to Africa. The older black inmate told the other ones to back off and slapped Billy in the face. This must have knocked some sense into him. He told him if he wanted to live another day in the cell he needed to go back in his bunk and not say another word. Billy sobered up enough to comply with this request.

After Janice made some calls, Billy was immediately transferred to the mental hospital for further care in Alexandria, LA. He was released after a few days and immediately went back to drinking. He had targeted a liquor store just outside of the base perimeter to steal from almost every day. When Janice and Lisa found this out, they both went to the management and begged them to prosecute Billy for stealing and they declined to do so! And once on the base, the military police would not prosecute Billy unless he actually committed a crime (of which being drunk and obnoxious was not one of).

BILLY

It soon got to the point where I got calls from Janice of how out of control Billy was and I had to call the base police to go to the house and handle it. At this point my feeling was to call the police EVERY time there was an incident so I could maximize the chances that no one would get hurt and maybe Billy could get into an institution where he would be forced to be away from alcohol.

Two weeks later Billy was again out of control enough to be hospitalized in Alexandria. While there, he decided to leave the facility and for a day he had an APB on him. I had made calls to the local police to look out for him because when in this state he could easily break into stores to steal more liquor. Who knows what he would do if he got desperate enough. They eventually ran him down a few miles from the hospital and placed him back in protective custody for another week.

While there he met Vanessa and Charlotte. Vanessa seemed like a very nice girl, 19 years old with a baby, but Charlotte was in the hospital because of multiple personality disorder. When Billy got out of the hospital, Charlotte took Billy on a wild ride to her house where they shot holes in the wall with the guns she had there, then went back to his room in New Llano. The next morning Charlotte's husband showed up at the door and he was a huge tree trunk of a man. Billy did not know Charlotte was married, much less left the address of his house on her kitchen counter! Janice calmed the husband down, and he explained Charlotte had done this constantly for the past year. She managed to get Charlotte out of Billy's room and into her husband's car while Billy stayed in his room and did not utter a peep. The husband was so nice about everything he actually stayed long enough to help find the house dog that had gotten loose!

During this time I was actually calling rehabilitation centers to see if they would take Billy, hoping that by the time I arranged something he would be ready to go. It was arduous work. I noticed that each facility was driven by what insurance would or would not pay. Despite the fact that I was able to get preapproval from our insurance company, I still saw lots of reluctance to take Billy out of fear they would not get paid. There were so many criteria to meet, I wondered some nights how anyone got accepted into a program any more.

A week before I came out to see them over Thanksgiving, apparently Billy got mad at a friend of his who owed him some money and in a drunken stupor he smashed the window of the parents' car in! This was a perfect opportunity to make Billy pay for his own foolishness I thought. Apparently not on an army base- the rule there is that the SOLDIER who is hosting the offender is responsible for any damage done on the base. So- my step-daughter was going to be stuck with paying for this damage even though SHE was the one who opened up her home to try to help Billy. Since she did this favor for us, we allowed her to repay a loan to us by paying for the window, which meant that we ended up paying for it.

I flew into Houston on November 23 and Janice and Lisa's neighbor picked me up. We all had Thanksgiving together in New Llano, and then all hell broke loose again. Apparently a friend of Lisa's accused Billy of touching Christopher inappropriately, and Lisa confronted him with it. Billy denied it and was furious, but before I could calm him down he punched a hole in her door. I was not hesitating to call the police anymore and immediately called them before the situation escalated even more. The police said that they had

BILLY

gotten way too many calls about Billy and he would have to leave immediately.

So in the middle of the night we left to find a hotel. Billy told us (truthfully) that despite his alcohol problem he would NEVER touch his nephew inappropriately. I believed that. Billy worried quite correctly that if he were jailed for this accusation he would be beaten in jail even before a trial was held. The next day they interrogated Chris for 10 hours and concluded that he was never molested and that Billy never did anything inappropriate with him.

We eventually landed in Alexandria, LA where again Billy was deciding not to go back to Virginia and face his capius. This time however, Janice WAS coming home as her staying with Billy to help him get his "act together" didn't seem to get him anywhere. So, this being his decision, we agreed to try to help. We got him a room at a local hotel- a weekly rate, and the desk clerk took a liking to Billy and agreed to help him find a job. We went to the grocery store and loaded him up for the week and wished him the best.

We knew there was a big chance Billy would go right back to drinking, but what else could we do? I was not quitting my job to follow an alcoholic around the country – and for what? It was time he got a little tough love- like all his probation officers and Loudoun County police had advocated for so long.

We left for home, and for the first week things seemed to be going well. Billy sounded good on the phone and told us of a couple leads he was pursuing for jobs. He reconnected with Vanessa who also lived in Alexandria and she told us she was going to do her best to help Billy stay clean.

The good feeling did not last. Two days after that phone call, we got a call from Vanessa. Billy had spent all his food money for the week on alcohol and pot, and then decided to steal beer from a local convenience store. After he got away with it the first time, he went back for more while the police were still there taking the report! The policeman just pointed for Billy to go straight into the police car for him to be taken to jail.

Billy was sentenced to 60 days in jail. Billy contacted a bail bondsman to bail him out and we said absolutely, unequivocally NO! Billy addiction was obviously out of control and since he didn't want to go to rehab, he was not going to go now. He was just going to have to pull the time.

At least Billy would be able to dry out some. He had come a long way from his "send the blacks back to Africa" speech and got really good at getting along with everyone. He became the clown of the Alexandria jail getting a laugh from everyone. He called home often, and we didn't realize until later that each call cost us $17 a call!

Initially the court told us that Billy could serve 60 days or pay a $460 fine, one or the other. Later, in late December 2003, the clerk of the court told me it was a day for day reduction of the fine. By this time, we were feeling a little bad that we left him in a jail by himself so far from home. Plus, it was a whole lot more convenient for me to pick him up at Christmas (when no one at the Government was working) that to do it at the end of January 2004. So, after Christmas we paid the remaining $230 fine (the phone calls alone would have cost us another $900 if we let him stay) and got him out on December 28, 2003.

BILLY

Chapter 17

2004. A new year brought new hope. That was good because we felt like we were running out of options. Billy was only 20 years old and I felt we were a bad decision or two away from losing him. We had booked a timeshare in Vero Beach, FL, and we thought Billy would appreciate a break from jail. Again, he still did not want to come back to Virginia to face the music, so we talked about him getting a place in Florida to try it again. This time, I was blatant about the fact that setting him up in a place of his own was doomed for failure. He was not ready. He needed to go to a halfway house or rehab, but unfortunately he already used up his rehab stay limit until July 1, 2004. We had some time to try to figure it out.

We picked Billy up from the Alexandria, Louisiana jail and headed to Vero Beach, FL. The honeymoon didn't last too long. When we got to Florida, Billy's addictions kicked in stronger than ever. I wondered if his 30 day hiatus did any good at all. We all at fun on the beach in the day, but at night he was prowling the beach for alcohol. He actually took our keys one night and drove the car drunk through the streets of Vero Beach!

After our vacation in Vero Beach, we spent a couple days in Palm Bay, FL at a hotel. Days seemed to be consumed with shopping for cigarettes and energy drinks. We naively thought if he had those things, we could forgo the alcohol and DXM. By early January, I had to return to work and Janice chose to stay with Billy in Florida to try to get him settled.

Janice and Billy found an inexpensive motel on US 192 to stay in, and Billy actually did get a job selling household cleaners door to door. Unfortunately, the group relied on drugging their salesmen up to get them to work longer! Billy's days of stumbling into the motel drunk or stoned after work were starting to mount until Janice had enough. She actually was going to leave him on the streets to fend for himself (as we had constantly been advised to do) because he refused to enter into CITA, a halfway house in Melbourne, FL, but at the last minute decided on her own to bring him back to Virginia.

I had never anticipated this. He was wanted in Virginia, and now he is coming back home. I felt like Billy went around the country from Cape Cod to Louisiana to Florida and now he was back in Virginia, wanted by the police and his addiction to alcohol was worse than ever!

Then, on the other hand, being wanted may be a good thing. If Billy got out of control, started breaking things or went back to trying to commit suicide, he would be out of commission for more than 3 days. Also, we would not have to argue and beg the authorities to take him- he had a warrant!

Before it was even February, Billy was caught stealing DXM at the local CVS. I said to myself, maybe this is for the best because I can't force him to go to rehab and if he is in jail at least he can't ingest any DXM or alcohol. The police took him into the magistrate's office, and amazingly he let him go with no bond! I argued with the magistrate, telling him how dangerous Billy had become and how his addiction was out of control. Finally, he relented and changed his mind and sent the police to get him, but Janice had already picked him up just before they came out.

BILLY

I thought- how could Loudoun County have a warrant on Billy, the police know it, and the magistrate let him go? He showed up for the hearing in court the next day and amazingly again the judge released him on personal recognizance and a promise to show up for a later hearing! I thought, did they lose the record that he had a warrant on him? I knew when Billy skipped out on the promise to appear that he would now be facing some serious jail time when he was finally caught.

Since 2002, all we heard from the police is to let Billy suffer his own consequences when he messed up. Here he did, and they had him in custody, and then let him go!

Janice took Billy to a new psychiatrist when he got back home. The new psychiatrist evaluated his meds, but also determined that Billy was critically addicted to alcohol, to the point where he would have dangerous withdrawals if we just cut his alcohol off cold turkey. At this point, Billy was consuming 120 ounces of alcohol a day. The doctor's plan was to wean him off of the alcohol 10 ounces a week to zero. While he was doing this, he needed to continue to attend AA meetings.

I thought this was a crazy idea, buying the alcoholic alcohol. But, everything else had failed miserably, and at least we had a goal of no alcohol at the end of it. I had my doubts about this working, and keeping a fugitive at my house, but what else was I going to do? I felt we only had so many chances to turn his life around and break this addiction and then he would be dead and it wouldn't matter.

The first few weeks the plan seemed to be working, mainly because 120 ounces a day is a tremendous level to start with. Along with that came babbling speech, food spills in his room and his constant badgering to get more alcohol. We steadily reduced his intake every week though until he got it down to 60 ounces, then we seemed to hit a wall.

In the meantime, we suffered through slurred speech, ranting and cussing on a daily basis. Strangely enough, Billy did manage to get a great job taking care of dogs at a kennel, and he really did make the most of it. He was working 30 hours a week, loved his job and brought in good money, and I was very proud of him. The owners at the Executive Pet Center loved him, but after 5 weeks they offered him a 70 hour/week job or no job, because they needed someone to stay over some nights to watch the pets. Billy didn't feel he was ready for 70 hours a week and I had to agree with him, so he reluctantly resigned.

We struggled to try to provide Billy with some meaningful activity. He met a girl named Tiffany who was kind of eccentric but enjoyed doing things with him. He seemed to regress to a child like state sometimes, and quite often invited over a 12 year old friend named Pookie and they took turns throwing bottles into a firepit and shouting "Rick James" from the Dave Chappel show.

Janice got Billy a video camera in hopes that it would serve as an outlet for his creativity. Unfortunately, Billy quickly turned it into the "jackass" show. He actually jumped into the middle of a frozen creek in the middle of February just so he could get the video (and almost froze to death). His favorite thing was to make members of the family mad and video them charging at him or hitting him. It got so bad I had to take the camera from him- and the "jackass" stunts stopped.

BILLY

By mid- May 2004, Billy seemed to hit a wall. He went to New York City with his new girlfriend, EJ, begging us to trust him. He had saved enough money from working at the thrift store to go. We let him go, but he quickly spent all his money on alcohol and was soon wandering drunk through the streets of NYC. I got a call when they finally made it back asking ME to drive to the middle of DC to pick him up from the train station- I told him no way. EJ used her last bit of money to get a cab back to our house. Somehow they made it back, but I knew this could not go on much longer.

That day came on 26 May, the day before Labor Day. Billy had had his ration of 60 ounces of beer, but at 10 pm he was ranting for more. He said he just wanted to drink more and we said no he had had his ration and that was it. Soon he went outside in the yard and kicked in the glass fish tank. He followed that up by ranting and trying to pull the basketball goal down in the driveway. After those antics, it was no surprise that the police were called. They came in the house and cuffed him for failure to appear and took him to jail.

Ultimately, the "weaning off alcohol" approach failed. An addict is NEVER going to quit as long has he has a supply of his drug. We learned from that failed experience, and it would never be tried by us again.

Chapter 18

As expected, when Billy made it to court, he was facing an angry judge. Billy had skipped town in September 2003 to flee to Louisiana, then failed to show up for a mandatory hearing on a theft charge in March 2004. The judge gave Billy the maximum sentence on his pending charges, and made him serve them consecutively, which is highly unusual. Billy had burned his bridges and now he was going to jail.

We had pledged no more lawyers. Paying for Billy's last lawyer practically broke us and in the end didn't seem to get us anywhere. Besides that, the lawyer said after 2003 that was it for him too. Billy was then assigned a court appointed attorney. This attorney impressed me immediately- he fought hard to get Billy a fair shake. When the verdict came down, I immediately requested that we appeal to circuit court to give Billy a chance to go to rehab again. Given the choice between rehab and jail, I was pretty sure he would pick rehab. As soon as our new insurance kicked in on July 1, 2004, we would be eligible to go. We found a place in Maryland called the rehab, and after we worked out all the details and made all the arrangements, the circuit court allowed him to be released for 30 days to attend rehab. Again we were hopeful that something would click.

After 30 days in jail, Billy was more than ready to go rehab. Being in Emmitsburg, MD, it was a quick drive to visit him on Saturdays. Every Saturday he seemed to be doing better, he certainly seemed to be getting something out of this rehab.

As the days went by, I was realizing I had asked the court for 30 days for Billy's rehab. It turned out the rehab

BILLY

program only lasted 28 days. The problem with that is that this meant that Billy would have to come HOME for a weekend and THEN we would have to get him to go BACK to jail. This meant there was a possibility he would run and we would have to somehow run him down to finish his term. I tried to do something about this but getting another court hearing to fix this was so difficult to get in time we just hoped for the best.

While at rehab, Billy completed his work and actually was part of a play on sobriety. He had his 21st birthday in rehab. There he also met Abbey, a young mother from Baltimore who really seemed to take to us. The counselors were concerned that Billy was spending more time paying attention to Abbey than the program.

When 28 days was up, I really considered getting a hotel out in the middle of nowhere so Billy would not be tempted to binge that weekend. I had to go on a business trip that weekend; Janice assured me that everything would be ok.

On Saturday I had a bad feeling something was not going right, and sure enough Billy had gotten drunk and she needed help with him. I took an early flight back and prayed that we would be able to hang on until Monday when he was due back at the jail. The next morning we went to church and took Billy, he got paranoid and asked to be taken home. When I did that, he combed the neighborhood and found someone who gave him a six pack and he was plastered by the time we got back from home. He was so drunk he turned over on his hamburger and just laid in mayonnaise. I called the police and begged them to take him to jail NOW and not make us try to drag a drunk tomorrow; they said that since he was drunk in his own house, they could not bring him in. So we just had to deal with it.

Now I was thinking, it would have been WORTH the hassle of trying to change the report date back to jail!

I had to be back at work on Monday, but I was tired of dealing with the "what if Billy runs" issue. If he ran, they would put a warrant out on him and he would be in jail that much longer. He surprised both of us by honoring his word and going back to jail without an incident.

Once back in jail on August 1, Billy spent a week in the drunk tank because the jail was overloaded. I was hoping that one of these times he would get the hint and REALLY try to quit. After a week, they shipped him down to Lynchburg until the end of his term on 8 November. Visitation was just once a week on Saturdays for 20 minutes. Billy liked it much better than the "dungeon" in Loudoun because it was a modern facility with good ventilation and plenty of space to move around. Janice and I took turns going down on Saturdays to visit him, he sure appreciated it. In Lynchburg they also let us send books to him from Barnes and Noble, so I sent him a new book every week.

I go back to the point that the Loudoun County jails were overcrowded. The county had finally commissioned the building of a new jail, but somehow they only got enough money to build a jail with the SAME capacity as the old dungeon. I wondered, how on earth did that happen? The population of the county was steadily growing, yet they build a new jail with the same capacity. What that means is that Loudoun County will continue to spend a fortune shipping inmates to other facilities at a cost of $126 a day, almost twice as much as it costs to house them locally. Since many of the inmates had mental health diagnoses and addiction problems, it seemed crazy that money for mental health

BILLY

services was being cut every year. This left the jails to act as de-facto mental institutions and rehab facilities, and the extent that they served in this capacity was increasing steadily! I knew for a fact that if long term hospital care was available for Billy and he could be made to go to it, he would not be in jail. Yet, there was no money for rehab services and the wait to see a county psychologist was an incredible 6 weeks! You wondered what it would take to make someone at the state AND county level realize that they could SAVE $126/day per patient if they could get appropriate treatment to these patients, who were NOT criminals and most likely would be law abiding citizens if they could control their addictions and/or their mental illness! We learned that the food they give the inmates is certainly not enough to fill up a 21 year old male. We made sure he had enough canteen money to eat well. Fortunately the phone calls were not near as expensive as they had been when he called from the Louisiana jail.

The calculation of time that needed to be served on Billy's sentence left a lot to be desired. All days served on a given charge should count toward a sentence, however we found that for some reason only the time from Jan 1, 2003 was counted toward the sentence! We told Billy's court appointed attorney and he did some research and found Billy had served a substantial amount of time towards this charge in 2002 also! Unlike most court appointed attorneys, this one vigilantly pursued the issue and got the release date reduced from January 15, 2005 to November 8, 2004. Again, this led me to wonder, how many other inmates are serving too much time because the release date calculated by the jail is not calculated properly? It was becoming obvious to me that those that did not have money got the short end of the justice stick. Were those that did the miscalculating admonished or give Billy's attorney an apology? Of course not, because again there was little accountability in the system.

I went to the Loudoun County jail website and found an interesting but scary article on inmate costs. The article was obviously directed toward "concerned taxpayers" and pointed out how inmates must pay $5 for Tylenol and $25 for a doctor visit. We thanked God for having the resources that allowed Billy to have enough food to eat, his proper medication and funds for doctor visits. Those with no money could APPLY for indigence, but that application could take up to 2 weeks to grant. In the meantime, the inmate with no money would get NO care no matter how urgent his need to see a doctor. I could not believe such a barbaric practice was carried out just to save a buck, when in fact the taxpayers were paying a HUGE price everyday because the jail could not house all inmates and they had to be shipped out to other jails at a premium price!

This "fee for medical care" policy came back to bite them the following year, when an inmate with no money came to the guards with a high fever begging to see a doctor. He was told to apply for indigence status, but he told them he could not wait he needed medical care immediately. They shipped him down to Charlotte Court House, VA ADC anyway, and the young man died along the way of a massive infection. Unbelievably, since the family did not sue the county, no action was taken at all and the practice remained in effect.

Fortunately for us, Billy learned how to get along with all the inmates, and stayed out of trouble until his release date on 8 November. Billy was glad to be out, and we again certainly hoped we could do something different to keep Billy away from drugs and on the way to a productive life.

BILLY

Chapter 19

I picked Billy up on 8 November 2004 and we went down to see my family in Richmond. I thought it was important to let Billy know that his family did not consider him a criminal and they still loved him and wanted to see him get better. The lunch went well, but unfortunately Billy went almost immediately back to DXM and alcohol. We had concluded that we needed to show some more tough love, so we made a rule- if Billy came back to the house drunk or high he was not going to stay in our house that night if we could help it.

We would not have to wait long. On the night of November 22, Billy came back to the house completely drunk and out of control. We called the warming shelter and since the temperature was less than 39 degrees, they were accepting people who did not have a place to stay. We got Billy in the car and took him up there to the middle of Leesburg, and after a little cajoling, got the director to take Billy for the night. Since it was 10 pm and freezing outside, we expected Billy would collapse in his sleeping bag and we would pick him up in the morning.

This did not happen. Billy later told us he left shortly after we drove away and went to the drug store nearby to steal Robotussin and DXM. He then tried to walk home as the snow started, but he went WEST instead of east. He got his boots wet so he took them off and started walking in his wet socks. He made it all the way to Purcellville along the Washington O&D trail before he knocked on someone's door because he was freezing. They called the police to help him, and the first thing the police did was try to bring him back to our house!

I could not believe the contradictions. Every time the police would come to the house, they would tell us that we really needed to evict Billy from the house. They implied that if we didn't do this, that we were just enabling him. He would either sink or swim on the street. Yet, when we made the hard choice of taking him out of the house when he was drunk, the first thing the police did was bring him BACK to our house in the middle of the night. The officers who advised us to just abandon him didn't talk to the ones who brought him back to our house. So much for enabling.

Janice and I were so exhausted that we didn't hear anything that morning. The police said they knocked and knocked but we didn't move. He eventually took him back to the shelter (where he belonged) and we eventually DID pick him up in the morning. Since we were late for Thanksgiving, we went straight to Richmond.

In December Billy got a call from someone he met in jail, James L. Billy had told us James was in jail for failing to pay his child support, but he was looking to get a job to catch up on his payments. He was an adamant ex addict and a devout Christian.

We agreed to let James spend the night and had a chance to talk with him. I have to admit he was very clean cut and polite and he sure could quote the Bible. The first night he volunteered to take Billy to an AA meeting and we cautiously agreed.

Billy and James got back home fine and said the meeting went well. Again he seemed like such a nice man and a good influence on Billy we agreed to let him stay another night.

BILLY

We left for church on Sunday morning, and when we came back our car and James were gone. He left a note that he was going to see his family, but it sounded fishy to me. He did not ask us if he could use our car that morning, he just took it while we were gone. After hearing nothing by 5 pm, I made some calls- one of them was to the men's shelter where he had been staying. I asked if they thought he could have stolen our car and I got chills down my back when the man I talked with said "That is what he does".

I immediately called the police to report our car stolen. I tried calling his sister and was informed that his mother spent her last dime sending him to rehab in the Northwest only to see him go right back to crack.

This was Janice's favorite car- a 1991 Nissan Pathfinder. Next call we got was from the Arlington police that they had found the car torched. A day later after an APB was put out for L, he gave himself up and was sent to prison for 4 years.
We were crushed. Fortunately, we had insurance, but he easily could have been chasing crack in the middle of DC with our son in the car! We found out later that he actually DID take Billy into DC to get crack, and Billy was scared to death he was going to get shot. He was so addicted he drove the car while smoking it!

We trusted Anthony and he went back to being a heavy pot smoker and taking off to DC. We trusted James the Bible scholar and the same thing happened. We felt like we were damned if we got someone to help Billy and damned if we didn't. Billy felt terrible about what happened, but apparently not bad enough to warn us what happened on Saturday (if we would have known James L. would have been out that night).

We replaced the car with a 2004 PT Cruiser and we were back to 2 cars before Christmas. The Nissan had 183K miles on it so we could not be but so upset, but again it could have been a lot worse. This put an end to trying to find a sponsor who could help Billy with his addiction and live with us.

I ended the year by talking to a friend of mine from college. We talked about family and honestly I was hesitant about sharing anything about Billy, after the "he just needs a good kick in the ass" speeches. I mentioned Billy was still struggling but we were still hopeful. She declared this must have come from a traumatic event in his childhood, I told her I didn't know of any. She then told me I needed to kick Billy out of the house immediately, and EACH of us needed to get our own therapist. The conversation ended abruptly, but it made me more determined to stick with Billy until we found something that worked. Advice from folks who had not lived through this seemed to be severely lacking even when the person giving it had their heart in the right place.

Janice, Billy and I watched the clock move us into 2005, hoping for the best.

BILLY

Chapter 20

One could reasonably wonder why we paid so much attention to what a police officer said or a probation officer said about the best way to handle our son's problems. Intuitively, the best person to work with would be his psychiatrist or psychologist. The problem was that, due to confidentiality rules, they could (and would) not talk with us much. The only people that talked with us at all about Billy were the police and probation officers, and they did it because they were forced to deal with him on a regular basis. Since nothing we were doing seemed to even slow down the DXM/alcohol addictions and control his manic behavior, we felt like we really HAD to consider SOMETHING that would help him and maybe even protect us at the same time.

Even when we went to the trouble to get Billy to sign releases, most psychiatrists and psychologists were reluctant to talk with us. The problem was that every day we were living in a powder keg, and if we had a heads up that he was again using, we could try to take some countermeasures. Honestly, I felt that the nightmarish life we were living every day really was not a concern to them especially when compared to how many insurance authorized visits were left and what balance needed to be paid. As time went on, a deep seated dread started emerging that no one was actually going to help and the scene was going to end with either Billy killing himself or killing us, and that scenario was really just fine with the others we were interacting with because it really didn't affect their life whether this happened or not.

In early February I started a new more demanding job assignment. This assignment was much closer to home, but my ability to handle Billy emergencies in the middle of the day was severely hampered. My new boss expected me at work by 8:30 am and gone at 5 with a half hour for lunch.. that was it. This is not a big deal for someone who didn't have a son who had been hospitalized 12 times by that point, but obviously it was for me. At my other position in McLean, I could take off for emergencies so long as I made up the time. The first day of work I was lectured for taking an hour off for a Northrop staff meeting- and the thought of a crazed call coming into the office would not be as easy to handle. I was sick of catering to Billy at that point- I had to go about my own way now- at least to a point.

Despite our best efforts, Billy started to slide again. My mother passed away in mid February, and I was visiting her in Richmond every weekend up until she passed away. After that Billy agreed to work at the thrift store with Janice, but only if he could get cash the same day. In March, Billy had a number of days where he wanted to go to Countryside shopping center to "look for a real job" and undoubtedly ask for "lunch money". I finally told Janice we could not keep doing this because all he was doing was spending it on alcohol.

As Billy's condition worsened, I felt like I had to try something desperate. I made up signs and passed them to all the local pharmacies and convenience stores with his picture asking them to please look out for Billy coming into their store- he is undoubtedly stealing from you. I urged them to call the police if he stole anything and report it. Some did not want to bother, but after listening they agreed to keep the picture and look out for him. This exercise was extremely embarrassing, but I felt like I had to do something to try to save his life.

BILLY

On Sunday April 4, 2005 Billy again had ingested 32 Coricidin tablets and was scared enough to come to us for help. We called the ambulance and had him rushed to the hospital to have his stomach pumped, and after that he voluntarily agreed to be TDOed. They sent him to Prince William Hospital this time, and they kept him for 6 days this time. Billy proposed staying with his sister again- this time she and her husband had moved to Hopewell, VA. It had been a long time since the accusations about Billy inappropriately touching Chris had come out, and clearly neither Lisa nor Todd believed that for a minute. We asked Lisa and Todd and they quickly agreed to Billy's idea because they needed someone to pick Chris up from school while they were both working. We agreed because... what else were we going to do? Let him come home and do this all over again?

Billy apparently thought he would be able to get away with drinking more at the Roberts house. By now, everyone knew how bad of an addict Billy was and was watchful. Within a week of being in Hopewell, he rode his moped drunk, abandoned the moped and could not find it again. I told him it would not be replaced.

While Billy was gone, I called the police in a "non-emergency" situation to see if we could put our heads together and head off some endless "criteria" questions next time Billy went manic. I also wanted to discuss the "eviction criteria" with them. The Loudoun police had always told me that if I ever wanted to have Billy removed; we had to go through an eviction process that would take at least 30 days. This of course would be totally useless to us- if he was violent or drunk I just needed him out of the house for a night! The Loudoun magistrate, on the other hand, told me that if Billy was over 18 and didn't pay rent, he could be instantly removed from the house. I relayed this to both parties- the police didn't want to talk to the magistrate, and the magistrate told the police they need to listen to a judge and not make their own damn call on this issue!

I set as a goal to elevate the issue so we could have a single resolution. I finally arranged for the Chief of Police to meet with the Chief Magistrate. Four days later I got a call from the Chief of Police- the magistrate was right in the state of VA, Billy could be evicted instantly. This was not just an exercise to get the two feuding brothers to come to a truce- I needed the police to enforce this the next time Billy came home drunk or violent!

In early May, Todd took Billy on a car ride after he came home drunk one night. He told him he was taking him to a gas station and abandoning him since he had forgotten to pick up Chris again. After Billy begged and pleaded, Todd told him this was just a test – NEXT time he was going to let him out of the car and he could walk somewhere.

Two weeks later, it happened. He got so drunk he collapsed over a fence. Todd got a call at work that no one had picked up Chris, he had to leave work early and get his son. He came home to see Billy over a fence, told him to get in the car and took him to a gas station and put him out behind the store.

Soon the store attendant called the police and the police arrested Billy for drunk in public then took him to St Mary's hospital in Richmond, where my mother had passed away 2 months earlier. We got a call when he was in the hospital he had a blood alcohol level of .38 (not .038), 4.5 times higher than the legal limit. The doctor said he was on the verge of alcohol poisoning!

BILLY

After examining him, they returned him to the police where they jailed him for a night. When he came to in a cell, he knew it was really bad. We picked him up in Richmond the next morning.

Lisa asked if I was mad that Todd did this. Not in the least. Billy needed this. He was not listening to anything, putting himself in danger day after day- he needed a wake up call- Todd did exactly what he should have done.

Believe it or not, after we picked up Billy, we went on a mini vacation in Williamsburg with Chris. Todd just told Billy the way it was going to be and by golly he stuck to his guns about it.

We started off the vacation by going to Wet and Wild in Williamsburg. When we got there, Billy wondered out loud why none of the girls his age looked at him. I told him his hair was a mess- long and stringy and in his eyes. Not attractive at all. When he looked around and realized it was true, he looked at me and said "OK Dad lets go get it cut". I didn't waste a minute and made a beeline to the barbers where they took a tremendous amount of hair from his head. Immediately he looked better! He got plenty of looks the rest of the day- and I started to see there was indeed some hope for this fella.

Naturally I was disappointed how the year had gone so far. Despite everything we did, Billy was still drawing himself back to DXM and alcohol and his bipolar disorder was far from under control. What does a family do when they are out of ideas? The answer- keep trying. What else can you do?

Billy had a large mole on the side of his face that was now infected. At the very least we could have that removed, and on July 1 he would again be eligible for insurance-covered rehab (that is WHY we changed plans!). He was already starting to slip back when we got his mole removed, but he was admitted to back to an Emittsburg, MD rehabilitation center on July 1.

Things were different than what we had seen in 2005. Billy said he did not see the attention given like was given the previous year. After just 10 days, Billy called me to tell me he was desperately sick. After all the "fake" sicknesses I had seen, I was skeptical. He told me he begged to see a doctor on Thursday, but he was told the doctor was not coming in until Monday and he would have to wait. Furthermore, if he WENT to an outside doctor, he would be released.

I called the rehabilitation center to ask if a nurse had examined Billy, and the counselor I talked to indicated that he thought Billy was just trying to get out of attending the program. Billy then called back and said "Dad, I am calling you to PLEASE take me to a doctor now. I am so sick I am getting delirious; I can't wait until Monday to see a doctor. Please help me!"

That was sincere enough for me. I called our insurance company who told me to immediately take Billy to a doctor no matter WHAT the rehab center said. Janice took off work to go get him, only to find him there staggering around with what seemed to be a 102 degree fever! Janice gave the nurse a piece of her mind and rushed Billy to a doctor in Frederick, MD. Billy also had a bad cough, and they diagnosed him with the early stages of bronchial pneumonia, a very contagious illness! The doctor said if he were forced to wait until Tuesday like the local nurse had told him his condition would have been very serious! Billy said others at the rehab had it also, but many were afraid to seek outside

BILLY

medical help in fear that they would be released too and possibly go back to jail.

We got Billy on antibiotics and fortunately he cleared up after a few days. What nerve of the rehab center! My son was at their facility and very ill and they refused to treat him until the next week! Plus, they had numerous participants there with bad coughs, possibly very contagious, and did NOTHING about it. I was wondering how they could even stay in business!

Back at work, I immediately made calls to the Maryland Health Department, who did not seem the least bit moved to take any action by my report. Initially, I could not even TALK to anyone about my son's condition until my son signed a Health Insurance Portability and Accountability Act (HIPAA) release and it was faxed back, which wasted several days. When I finally could talk to someone at the health department, they told me they would not even do an investigation because they had been to the rehab a week earlier and didn't notice anything strange! I told them that was FAR from an investigation, they need to TEST the patients there with bad coughs (there were many) and find out how many had a contagious illness! Again I was stalled by more requests for more releases, and by the time I sent them in, NO ONE from the Maryland Health Department would return my calls. The claim was that if Billy was concerned HE should make the calls, but having just been released from doctors he was in no condition to do anything. Bottom line- the Maryland Health department was too lazy to bother with the situation. Again- no accountability that I could find.

In the process of making the calls to the Maryland Health Department, my boss called me in his office and warned me that I need to be doing work at work and not personal things. As any parent of someone who is bipolar and a chronic addict, there are things that you just have to handle and most of them will not wait until you are off work. Furthermore, the things that will wait can't be handled because THEIR business hours are 9 – 5 pm. Finally, Janice was not in a position to make these calls because she was busy moving Billy into his new place in Frederick, MD!

I apologized and explained about our life with Billy. My boss apologized and was very sympathetic, but asked that I use HIS office to handle any Billy related emergencies because I could then close the door (my office was in a cubicle outside his office). I told him that I would do what I could to minimize this, but that there probably would be a fair share of emergencies I would have to handle in the middle of the day. Since no cell phones were allowed in the building, I probably would need to use the phones to handle emergencies from time to time. I wish my life was different, but these were the cards I was dealt and I have no choice but to play them. Fortunately, my boss accepted that and pledged to work with me.

After Billy was released from rehab, I had told him he was not coming back to live with us. It wasn't working. He wanted to try living on his own. Remembering the disaster in Alexandria, LA, I didn't have a lot of confidence it would work. But what else could we do? We were not sending him to rehab where with other people with infectious conditions go untreated. We agreed to put Billy up at a hotel in Frederick, MD temporarily until we could find a halfway house or some inexpensive housing he could live in.

We checked him in a motel and found the nearest AA meetings to him. We decided if we were going to start

BILLY

him out in this new town he wanted to move to, he needed some start money. I got him a Mastercard where I was the primary cardholder and the limit on the card was $300. We stayed the weekend with him, walked him to his AA meetings, and found a few places he could see if they needed help at. The halfway house in Frederick worked in conjunction with The Good Shepherd, but they were still full when Billy was there.

We bought him some groceries for the week then returned to Sterling hoping for the best. Billy abused the card in the first 3 days, so I called Mastercard and had it suspended. Other than that, he did OK and attended his AA meetings every day (they were in biking distance). I visited him the following weekend and we even went swimming together at a public pool.

Making it two weeks was too much to ask for I guess. In the middle of the week, we got a call from a massage therapist who was staying at a hotel that Billy was so drunk he could not stand up. We called the local hospital and sure enough he was there with a blood alcohol level of .39! We went to get him, and found that there is no drunk in public law in the state of Maryland! They took him to the hospital merely because he was a threat to die. Once they confirmed that he was not going to die, they were ready to release him to the street!

This state was worse than Virginia, if that is possible. We first went to the hotel and cleaned out his room, got his bike, then picked him up. I remembered that .39 was considered to be the level alcohol poisoning occurred. On the way back, we called Janice K. She felt a calling to set up a home for recovering addicts in Leesburg and secured federal money to do just that! An opening became available on August 1, and for $200 for the month, Billy moved in. We figured that he would be living with other people who would keep an eye on him, and we would be closer. Again we bought Billy some groceries and hoped for the best.

BILLY

Chapter 21

I think at that point Janice and I were just fooling ourselves because we needed a break from the havoc that Billy would cause if he were living at home. Also, since he just got deathly ill after going to a rehab where no one cared to stop the illness from spreading, I didn't see how that would help him. This new "halfway house" seemed to be as good as any place for Billy to hang his hat on.

We told the procurer Janice K about Billy's alcoholism, and we told everybody else in the house about it and to keep an eye on him. That was one big reason he was there. The first day he got one of the young ladies in the house to take him up to the grocery store and came out with a gallon jug of wine! I asked first – why did you let him buy that and second- how on earth did he pay for it? She gave a lame excuse that "she didn't know Billy was an alcoholic" and told me he paid for it with a credit card his Dad gave him. I thought to myself- that is impossible- I suspended that card a week ago. But where was he getting his money?

I called Mastercard just to make sure it was still suspended. To my horror, I found that they allowed Billy to activate it again! When I set up the card, I specifically made it so he could NOT activate it- only I could! I told them to immediately terminate it FOREVER. They apologized and did not bill me for what was charged, but the damage was done- he got almost a week's worth of alcohol with it.

At the two week mark, I got a call while I was at work. Billy had drunk so much he was crawling on the floor and cussing at everyone. Janice called our pastor to help and Billy proceeded to cuss him out, so the police were called. Billy was claiming since we paid his rent for the month, he could do anything he wanted. Not so- we did this so he would clean up and get better not get out of his mind drunk. The police were called to evict him and he was eventually TDOed. This time his blood alcohol level registered .38, and the examining doctor told us his prognosis was poor.

I found out there was a new wrinkle added to the TDO criteria in 2005. NOW apparently if someone made a suicide threat when they were intoxicated it didn't count. ????? Apparently one needs to WAIT while the person sobers up to see if they repeat the threat and HOPE they don't actually kill themselves while we are waiting for that to happen. And of course, if they ACTUALLY commit suicide they DO meet criteria. That was reassuring! I am sure the new wrinkle was added to again REDUCE the number of patients that are actually TDOed as the mental health budget was again reduced.

Here Billy was, 22 years old and he was on the verge of having a stroke because he had abused his body so bad. We knew things were getting desperate and we had to step in to try to save him or he would be taken away in a body bag. I kept thinking- he is way too young for this- my son is going to die in front of me and I am just watching it happen. Not if I could help it.

BILLY

Chapter 22

This time when Billy was released, we took him back home. Yes we had a rule about not taking him home, but I was not going to put him somewhere else and watch him die either. Obviously he was not capable of making it on his own. As expected, his addiction started back by the second day home in August 2005.

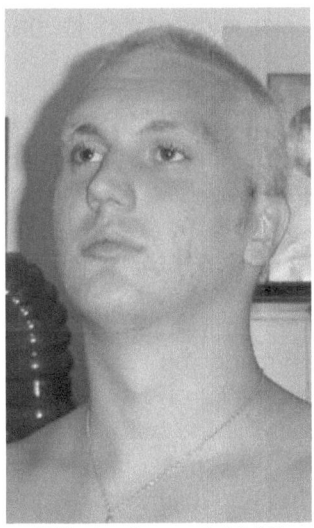

Billy in August 2005

At this point, I started again looking for another rehab. What else were we going to do? I called the LAMPS (Loudoun Adult Medical Psychiatric Services) program at Loudoun County Mental Hospital in hopes of them having a program that Billy could go to in lieu of a TDO. The attending nurse answered the phone, and told me she remembered Billy.

She told me that the program would not be open to someone who just wanted to check in. She went on to say that maybe the best thing for Billy is to just abandon him in Leesburg. That way he would either sink or swim. She had actually done that with her son and he straightened himself out.

I thought- what a crazy piece of advice! Without meds or a home, Billy would almost CERTAINLY die- after he robbed all of local pharmacies of their DXM products! And if he did, the nurse who gave this advice would not care- it would be just another day for her. WE would be affected the rest of our lives. For what- so our lives would be easier??? For me, I would rather have a hard life with a chance that my son could recover than an easier life with him out of it. I think any loving parent would feel the same way.

Again, if my son had a broken leg, NO ONE would suggest I abandon him in Leesburg to fend for himself as maybe he will straighten himself out. If this lady had her son clean himself up on his own after being abandoned, he is a lucky one – a rare one. Billy clearly was not happy with his life but obviously could not stop the addictions on his own. Morally, I owed to Billy to keep trying to help him while also trying to keep my own sanity- which by the way was getting harder to do every day.

In October 2005 Billy relapsed and in the middle of a football game he told us he had taken 64 Corocidin tablets. Now we were going back to DXM! We rushed him to the hospital, hoping he would not die on the way. The doctors immediately tried to pump his stomach, but he pulled out his IVs and was trying to break out of the hospital. The doctor their ordered a medical TDO (this was a first for Billy) so they could restrain him and pump

BILLY

his stomach. They did that successfully and took him to the hospital for assessment, where they then gave him a psychiatric TDO for 3 days and sent him back to LAMPS.

While there, Billy was assigned another doctor. The doctor let it be known immediately that he didn't want to speak to us, just Billy. He let Billy talk him into prescribing him Adderall again. The last time Billy was prescribed (non-time release) Adderall he went out of his mind and was picked up in Richmond, VA. The doctor did not want to hear about any of Billy's history with medication. Again, the fact that Billy was willing to sign a release didn't change the doctor's stance.

Apparently the Adderall was fueling Billy's addiction to DXM again. Although we did have a fun father and son weekend at the end of October in King George, the good times were not to last. On Saturday evening November 5th I went to our girl's end of the season softball team party, and when I came back I found the house in complete darkness. I heard Janice call me from the neighbor's house; apparently Billy had gone completely out of his mind and was threatening her and talking like Satan. She had called the police, I checked out the house to find that Billy had left the house. We pleaded with the police to search for him as he could have been in the process of killing himself now, they responded magnificently by sending out a full squad to look for him- officers, dogs and a helicopter! Billy managed to elude them all night while staying in the neighborhood, hiding in the creek bed, walking through apartments and leaving his footprints then going the other direction, etc. The police finally stopped him in the woods across the street but he bolted from them and leaped down a 20 foot embankment onto the rocks and kept running.

Woody Hawthorne

The police told me at midnight they had 4 good charges on him- that was fine with me I just wanted him confined somewhere before he killed himself or someone else! One officer waited until 1 am then left- and Billy showed up an hour later, smirking that he eluded the entire Loudoun County police squad. I called the police back at 6 am when Billy was asleep, but amazingly they said that NOW they had no charges on him and could not arrest him.

I thought- how could this be? How could a charge "go away" after a few hours? How could he be rewarded from escaping the police? Now Billy was smirking and cocky- I knew this would not be the end of it. He actually said the whole evening had been like an adventure!

That morning Billy admitted that the Adderall was making him crave DXM like never before- and this was driving him. I wanted to really "thank" the new doctor for that one! We flushed the rest of the Adderall. Billy had dangled out to us he needed it to "study and read" again but I never saw him do either when he had it!

Sure enough, two days later on Monday, I came home to find Billy in his "DXM" trenchcoat, a glazed look and a nasty attitude. He declared he was going for a walk- I knew that meant he was going after more DXM. I walked with him down the road on a freezing night, then he started sprinting down the street into the woods. I ran with him, then he wandered to picnic area at Broad Run Farms. He stripped down to his underwear and started growling. I had seen enough and went home to call the police.

So within a few minutes we had another search party, dogs and helicopters. I kept thinking- if they would have

BILLY

picked him up on Saturday we would not be going through this again! The police searched for 6 hours until midnight and again gave up, this time they waited down the street. When Billy saw the last squad car leave from in front of our house, he walked back in and made his way to the second floor. I begged him to voluntarily to go the hospital for a TDO, he refused. Then without warning he bolted towards the living room window as if to leap out from the second floor. I stopped him and the fight was on. I restrained him and Janice grabbed his legs and held them. He had tremendous strength and it was all I could do to hold him down. Janice finally tied his feet and managed to call the police from the cell phone and let the police 2 doors down know where we were.

It seemed like an eternity, but the police finally made it up the stairs and shackled him. I was exhausted. Like us, the police were frustrated in continuing to go through these takedowns only to see him released after 3 days and doing this all over again. The officer gave me a look and asked me if I had been assaulted during the fight, and I remembered he hit me with a vase from the coffee table. Wanting Billy to be confined for more than 3 days, I said yes he did assault me. An assault charge would put him in jail for a few more days at least and he would only be released under a slew of conditions- and he had no conditions now.

He was arrested and taken to jail, but the police forgot to TDO him first! Anyway after 5 days the judge released him after they gave him a no contact order for me- we got him a room with friend Stan and they stayed there for a few days. His hearing was set for mid December, so with a no-drinking clause in his release conditions, we took him back.

I was desperate to find some answers to all of this. I again tried to engage the services of a new counselor- this time we tried a lady psychologist who worked in Countryside right up the road from us. Billy had gotten obsessed with moving to Amsterdam and getting a flat- obviously he read that it was legal to buy drugs there. He was looking up plane tickets on the internet.

The three of us went to the new licensed in-network psychologist and honestly we were not impressed. We had her talk to Billy who told her his objective in life was to watch DVDs and go to Amsterdam. He didn't have any skills or plan he just wanted to go. He then excused himself, and she talked with us. First, she didn't say anything about Amsterdam because she didn't want to "burst his dreams" (she was leaving that to us because we sure were not going to let him go). Second, she recommended I get a "babysitter" for Billy because my wife was going to be too stressed leaving him on his own ever.

A babysitter for a 22 year old man. That was the most ridiculous and impractical thing I had ever heard. First of all, you could not even HIRE someone to babysit a 22 year old man 24/7. Second, Billy would slip away from him just like he slipped away from Janice even when she quit her job to stay home with him. Did anyone think that maybe Janice could learn to live her own life and just seize the chance to get him help when we could? After that, I thought maybe I should go back to the police and the probation officers for advice. Did we just pay this woman $150 per hour for this advice????

While at home, Billy looked like he was trying to be good, but was struggling every minute. We had taken away his moped because he had broken the chain on it

BILLY

when I had locked it previously. This time I took it to work behind a chain link fence.

This time Billy had a new male probation officer while awaiting trial. At this point, I told Billy that he needed to go BACK to rehab or go to jail. I took several nights of research, insurance calling, bed checking etc. of the nearest rehabs and found one in Shippensburg, PA- the Roxbury Treatment Center. We noticed that now 30 day programs were on the "outs" because insurance would not pay for them. The most we could get was 10 days- better than nothing. After arguing for several days with the insurance company about what constituted "days used", they agreed to pay for treatment.

In early December when we drove him there, we AGAIN were arguing with the insurance company. The insurance company told Roxbury that Billy was NOT approved for treatment, even though I got this all squared away before we left Leesburg. While this was going on, Billy was showing signs of refusing to check in. After 3 hours we FINALLY got the insurance company to honor its promise AND we got Billy to agree to enter treatment rather than go right back to jail. We left him there at 5 pm and drove home exhausted.

At 10 pm we got a call from Billy. He left treatment and now he was freezing in the street. I was so mad. I thought about picking him up the next day, but if he froze to death that night (it got down to 14 degrees) I would never forgive myself. We got back in the car and drove 3 hours back to Shippensburg to pick him up. By this point, I knew his new PO would revoke his bond (he got the bond from the magistrate SO he could go to treatment) and get back to jail. The problem was that the bond revocation was not instant- he had to submit a recommendation that the bond be revoked and WAIT for a judge to get around to doing it- and that could be days. So now we had to keep him from creating an incident for a few more days.. THAT was going to be a challenge.

BILLY

Chapter 23

Janice and I knew he had an order and he broke it. We also knew that a probation violation would have to be reported to a judge, a judge would EVENTUALLY consider the request and then action might be taken. If Billy went manic, we needed something the police could act on quickly.

We remembered that a week earlier Billy had broken our safe to try to get to his meds. I remembered that- so if Billy was out of control we could get him off the streets immediately. We didn't need to wait long. On Friday December 16th Billy came in drunk after a night at the Eight Ball bar and wanted to start a fight. We now got to the point that as SOON as we saw trouble, we called the police. They came over and did a breath test on him to find he had a .06 blood alcohol. For someone who has a probation order not to drink ANY alcohol, that is a violation. Just as I suspected, the police would not take him in on that NIGHT, again waiting for a judge to give an order. We knew that meant days more of arguments and drunken nights, so I told the police of Billy's vandalism on the safe. This was my ace in the hole. At first there was some debate on whether they could consider a charge that was 2 weeks old, but thank goodness they did. Billy was so upset with the charge that he verbally abused the officers all the way to the magistrates' office. They put him in jail with no bond, and immediately considered his failure to observe the probation rules to revoke his probation. Billy would now be in jail for a while.

We were not thrilled with the way we had to get Billy away from DXM and alcohol, but it did the job. He was safe at night and not ingesting anything but food and water every day. Janice and I took the opportunity to take a vacation from the insanity so we headed down to Cocoa Beach, FL for the holidays. We were starting to learn to take advantage of these breaks to recharge our batteries for the next round. We so appreciated a quiet night free of wondering what Billy was getting into. We enjoyed the trip, and Janice again suggested that I submit my resume to the Northrop Grumman facilities down here to see if they needed an EMI engineer. The Northrop Grumman Integrated Systems in Melbourne, FL was closed over the holidays, but there was a guard available at the front gate to take a resume. To my surprise, they were in a hiring mode at that time and I got a call to come down for an interview when I got back. I had a great interview on 24 January, and waited to see what was to come.

Billy was released from jail in mid January 2006. The first weekend back me, him and his friend Derrick went paintballing and had a great time. Billy always enjoyed that, and he was good at it. Plus, while we were paintballing he was not thinking about drugs.

The following week was a different story. He asked if he could have his moped back one morning, I told him he was a long way from earning it back yet. So he asked if he could use my skates to get some exercise- I should have known better. He used them to skate 5 miles up to the Giant, outside of the area of stores where I had passed out his picture.

When I talked to the manager later, I found that Billy cased the store like a pro and waited for the girls at the register to take a break then he made his move. When he was caught at the door he pushed his way past the employees with bottle in hand and ran- leaving my skates behind. The store never pressed charges or

BILLY

even notified us even though they indeed had the poster I had left to them from 2004.

Meanwhile, Janice and I continued to struggle to deal with this week after week, month after month. We managed to find a great support group that met in Leesburg on Saturday mornings. Lots of good people with lots of good experiences and ideas. Most importantly, we all gave each other hope!

Since he had also gotten drunk another time that week, I called his probation officer. All he was doing was leaving each day and getting drunk- he again needed to be off the streets. I called his new PO on 26 January 2006, his probation officer. When I finally reached her, she was in a foul mood. She made it clear earlier that she didn't like to talk to parents and clearly felt that Janice and I were just "enabling" him to misbehave. When I reached her, I told her he again drank this week and begged her to violate him so he could get off the streets. Another day like this and we could easily wake up to a dead Billy. Then she told me "You know what? Maybe it would be better for everyone if the next time he attempted to commit suicide you should just not call the police and let him die. I know that would be hard for you and your wife to do, but maybe it would be for the best."

I hung up on her. That was unbelievable. She must have felt pretty confident there were no consequences for saying anything she felt like for her to say that. No it would not be better if we just "let him die". It would be better to fight like hell to get him better than to waste a human being and let him die because he was a burden to the system. Again, if Billy died, it wouldn't bother her a bit; in fact I am sure she has forgotten all about who Billy Hawthorne is now that he is not on her caseload. Janice and I, on the other hand, would NEVER get over him passing away. I think I did what any parent would have done and would continue to do- fight like hell to save their son.

I called the next day to her supervisor to complain and left a message, and I got no call back. My expectations were low at that point. I half expected the supervisor to say "what about what she said didn't you understand?" I would call both of them later and leave messages, but it would take another year before I finally would get a response. In 2008 I finally got the supervisor to return my call, and at that time he claimed the PO vehemently denied saying that, but I know what I heard. It was easy for me to see that Community Corrections really didn't care what their employees said- because there was very little accountability of anyone's actions to anyone else.

Since the following week was rough, I asked him if he wanted to have a friend Derrick over again and he said sure. This time, things did not go so easy. He wanted to go see a movie, and he had a bad attitude.

Billy found a movie he liked, and then demanded that I take him an hour earlier. Given his reputation for stealing Robotussin, I told him I would get him to the movie in time for the movie and no earlier. While I was in the bathroom, he and Derrick then called his mother who was working and asked if she could drive them to the movies! I intercepted the call and told her I was taking them at the proper time and no one was going to bother her while she was at work.

Billy then announced he was walking to the movies, and walked around the block twice and came back in time for me to take him myself. Something was not right, but I had hoped since Derrick was with him he would stay out of trouble.

BILLY

Again, not to be. Around 6 pm, it started snowing and we got a call from CVS. They caught Billy stealing Corocidin tablets again. He put the packs in his backpack and the alarm went off as he was taking off. The attendant recognized who it was from the posters I had left earlier. I BEGGED them to please press charges before he again overdosed on them. The lady told me it was a pain to do that, but since I had asked her she agreed. Apparently Billy went in after the movies with Derrick intending on stealing them whether Derrick was with him or not. When Derrick saw this, he offered to BUY Billy the Corocidin but Billy insisted on stealing them- a matter of pride he said. The police were called while Billy was walking back in the snowstorm and they picked him up for shoplifting. So on January 28 his personal recognizance bond was again revoked and again he was left to detox in the drunk tank.

Meanwhile, I had accepted Northrop's offer to transfer from Information Technology to Integrated Systems in Melbourne, FL. I was thrilled. I got to keep all the salary I had up in Northern Virginia while still being able to move to a state with a lower cost of living and no income tax! Plus, I was going to be doing engineering work and getting away from systems integration and note taking in a super classified environment. Finally, we could get Billy OUT of Loudoun County and the state of Virginia, with the hope that mental health patients would be treated better in Florida. Janice and Billy had urged me to move back to Florida every year for the last 10 years, so not surprisingly they were both thrilled. Now all we had to do was sell the house.

Back in Virginia, Janice and I both felt it was time to try rehab for Billy again. We had tried many times obviously, but we felt like our best chance for him to break this cycle of addiction was to keep getting treatment. One of these times something might click- it was certainly not going to click in jail. We found a place in Salisbury, MD called the Hudson Center that looked promising, and they accepted our insurance. They also had a bed opening up when we inquired in March 2006. Given this, we again went to the Circuit Court and asked for Billy to be released to attend treatment at the Hudson Center. Billy's court appointed attorney did a great job working for us to frame a plan that a judge would accept. In a March hearing, the Circuit Court judge granted Billy's request to attend treatment in Salisbury, MD- and a warning that if he DID NOT complete his treatment that he would be returning straight to jail.

The judge granted the request, and on Monday 27 March I picked Billy up from jail and took him straight to Salisbury, MD. Part of the conditions for release was complete and immediate payment of court costs. I thought it was interesting to note that the entire 4 years we were dealing with Billy's mental illness and addictions we were CONSTANTLY told by the police and the probation officers that we needed to STOP helping ("enabling") Billy, yet when it came to collecting THEIR money, they insisted on us "helping" him by paying all costs immediately before he could be released. We remembered the same thing when the police would pick him up drunk, they immediately took him back to OUR house and dumped him off in our front lawn and took off. Moral philosophies were only useful so long as THEY were not stuck with the problem.

Billy checked into Hudson House on Tuesday, 28 March. I joked with Billy he missed the final week of March Madness- which was his least favorite TV entertainment. Billy did well at the Hudson House at

BILLY

first, then we got word that Billy was on the verge of being kicked out of the program. We asked Hudson House why, they could not tell us because of confidentiality rules. We called our insurance company, we were told the same thing. I thought if the insurance company had miscounted eligible days, we needed to find this out and fix the problem. We didn't not know what the insurance company was telling Hudson House, but to head off a problem I calculated his allowable days of treatment and sent it to our insurance company, asking them not to terminate treatment because he was out of insurance coverage.

To find out what was going on, I had to fill out a waiver for Billy to sign, have him sign it, fax it to us so we could fax it to our insurance company while Hudson house also kept a copy for themselves. That whole process took 3 long days. When we finally found out what was going on, it turned out Billy was not completing his assignments and THAT is why they were ready to kick him out. Fortunately, he had turned things around and really seemed to be getting something out of the program. By the time we visited him on Saturday, he was in good standing. He had great counselors, and really seemed to be changing his attitude. Billy completed his program successfully in 17 days, and we picked him up and brought him home on 14 April. He had a very good attitude and I felt confident if I could just get him out of his familiar environment we would have a better chance of keeping him on the right track. I told Integrated Systems I would be able to report to work in Melbourne FL on 31 May. We had cleaned and polished the house up for sale, and things were indeed looking up.

Chapter 24

On Monday April 17, 2006 we let Billy's girlfriend he met at the Loudoun hospital the previous year, Jenny, come over since he had been so good that previous weekend. It was a rough one because our cat of 12 years, Cinnamon, had just passed away in our bed. At 5 pm, I stopped at the Home Depot on the way home to pick up some more paint stripper to get up some remaining paint spots in the living room- so the house would look perfect for potential buyers.

I got home at 5:30 and the house was empty. Plus, the white pickup truck was gone. This was a truck a friend of mine Tina had given Billy, but since it was a shift car, he didn't want anything to do with it. In fact, he told me that if it were up to him he would drive it off a cliff. Janice took it over and we got it fixed up and used it to move big items when we needed to- it was nice to have. But- it was gone AND Janice's PT Cruiser was gone. Just as I was wondering what the heck was going on, a police officer showed up at the door and told me that Billy was in a car accident at Countryside.

I thought- what car was he in? I called Janice on the cell phone, and she explained that Billy had gotten into some liquor and he was being belligerent. He tried to take his moped, but she was able to get to it first to lock it up. Janice then took Jenny home and left Billy there. Apparently, Billy decided to root through the house and find the keys to a shift car he didn't know how to drive and somehow cough and sputter his way up to the Countryside shopping center where he ran into the back of another motorist.

BILLY

After he ran into the back of the other car, Billy himself hit his head and was dazed. He ran over to a phone to call Janice who took him back to the scene right away. He got there 26 minutes after the crash and was promptly arrested by the officer on the scene.

I could not believe it. I was disgusted- and still could not believe he made it up to Countryside without stalling! He NEVER drove that car one time over the entire year we had it- and never had any interest in driving it. It was like we knew that sooner or later something bad was going to happen if he continued nursing his addictions, and it did.

Based on what we had seen before, even if I had gotten home before he took off, the police STILL would not have detained him because he was drunk in our house and he didn't meet the criteria of being picked up. Billy was taken to jail and we were in no way inclined to bail him out.

Billy's bail was set at $2000 and he was sent to Blue Ridge Detention Center in Lynchburg, VA until his trial for drunk driving. Lynchburg he where he served the last part of his 2004 sentence. After talking to him there for several weeks, he asked for the chance to go to a halfway house so he could show the judge that he was starting to get his life together before his trial. Otherwise, he was facing jail for a long time with no mental health care. We talked to the folks who were in charge of the local men's shelter in Loudoun (that is what Good Shepherd Thrift Store supported) who told me that they had one opening there, but Billy had to report there before Monday May 8th. If we waited until they brought him back up to Loudoun on Wednesday the 10th, the opening would be given away. After some consideration, I drove down to Lynchburg on Sunday May 7 and bailed him out.

When I got him back up, the OTHER director of the shelter told us there were no more openings! Obviously there was a communication breakdown, and now we had Billy out and there was no shelter opening after we had been promised one before I went down to get him.

After we got word that Billy could not get into the local men's shelter, I spent hours calling other shelters from other localities like Winchester, Manassas, etc. I ran into the same objections- there were a ton of requirements, not any available beds, and policies that did not accept people that were out of their county. I told them OUR County didn't sponsor ANY men's shelters! Frustrated I breathed a big sigh and hoped for the best.

Surprisingly, Billy did not go straight back to DXM and alcohol. He had made a pledge to stop before he killed someone, and he was putting all his willpower into doing just that. Thankfully, there were no more incidents before I had to leave for Florida at the end of May. I had hoped to take Janice and Billy with me, but unfortunately the house was not even close to selling.

I believe this was the time Billy started his schizo-affective behavior. He had become one with a Native American spirit, Chief. He was trying hard to keep it together, but felt moved to build memorials to the spirit and play with his dog Harvey. Harvey was half lab and half chow and Janice and I got him in December 2005 when he was a pup. His mother was rescued from a rooftop during hurricane Katrina, and she had 9 puppies after she was rescued, with Harvey being the runt.

BILLY

Harvey really seemed to keep Billy busy. He did have a few slips while I was gone, but he worked hard to stay clean. For the most part he was successful. Billy and Janice came to visit me in Florida in the middle of July, and it was good to see them. The first day after I picked him up from the airport, he asked me to take him and get a tattoo. Since he seemed to be doing better, I did that. But later that night he met up with a guy who had a stripper for girlfriend, and he needed a ride. I could not keep up with him anymore by 11 pm and we went to bed. I found out later he had stolen $20 from my wallet and drank with the hotel guests all night.

By morning he was so drunk we had to call the police to get him out of the room. Another ugly scene that resulted in him being escorted out. At this time, they could not take him in for being drunk. An hour later we had a bad feeling and went on the beach to find him because lying down in the heat with that level of blood alcohol was dangerous. We found him passed out with the surf lapping at his heels and people stepping over him to get around him. He was in bad shape. I pulled the car up to the beach and Janice and I lifted him into the air conditioning and gave him some Gatorade. His eyes were in back of his head and he looked like he was near death.

As disgusted as I was about him being drunk, I was not about to let him die. We considered taking him to the hospital, but I didn't want to argue with hospital attendants on whether or not he met criteria for being admitted! We moved AWAY from the beach and got a place in Palm Bay for the rest of the trip. Thankfully we had no more drinking incidents for the rest of the trip. Billy met a girl at a seafood restaurant and they decided to go the beach that night to see the sea turtles lay eggs. At 11:30 pm Billy asked to use my keys to get something in my car, but I was afraid he would lose my keys so I just gave him my remote.

When Billy got back, he said he had a neat time but alas he lost my remote to my car. Since they are expensive to replace, I drove to Sebastian Beach where he saw the turtles to look. At that point, Billy really seemed to lose it. He was wild eyed and digging dramatically into the hermit crab holes looking for the remote. After an hour I told him we need to give up and got him a Gatorade. On the way north he kept going on and on how he knew everything about physics and actually knew just about everything there is to know.

A few days later we moved to a Days Inn where Billy managed to capture an iguana with the help of 6 other kids at the pond he had spent a lot of time as a child. When it was time to fly back on 27 July, we had problems. On the morning of the flight, Billy declared that he was not going home. He had charges to face, and if he didn't go back for them he would be guilty of a felony and an APB would be put on him. He planned to "live off the land" in Palm Bay with the homeless people.

After an hour of arguing, I finally convinced Billy to fly back for his hearing, and he and Janice just made it to the Orlando airport to catch their plane home. When Billy went to his hearing, his court appointed attorney did manage to settle his DUI with time served and a fine – she did a great job. Earlier, the district attorney had heard from the victim of the car wreck who pressured him into charging him with a felony.

He was able to come up with hit and run. After Billy crashed the car, he hit his head and ran to a phone to call his mother, but was back at the scene 26 minutes later and was not charged with hit and run at the time.

BILLY

Weeks later, the district attorney managed to find a policeman who was not at the scene at the time to declare that Billy had been away from the scene for more than 2 hours, which I immediately said was baloney and we would fight it. At the court appointed attorney's urging, Billy agreed to be TRIED for this, but I was confident with the right investigation he would be acquitted.

Apparently the district attorney took this as an AGREEMENT to plead guilty to a felony. Not the case at all. Since Billy's court appointed attorney seemed anxious to put the deal to bed, Janice and I both agreed it was time to hire Billy his own attorney. It so happened that Billy's old court-appointed attorney in 2004 was now in his own private practice and available to represent him - so we hired him.

Billy's new private attorney immediately went to work. He made clear to the district attorney there was NO written plea agreement from Billy, and there was going to be no guilty plea. Also, he found out the policeman who claimed Billy was away from the accident scene for two hours was not even AT the scene, and was making up the story about Billy being missing from the scene. Billy deserved punishment for running into the back of a car, but he didn't need an officer to lie about what happened to get him there. Billy's attorney FOUND the officer who was on the scene and that officer courageously told the truth that Billy returned to the scene 26 minutes after the crash, contradicting the other officer who invented the story that Billy was away from the scene for 2 hours. God bless him. Did that original officer face any consequences for lying about Billy being gone from the scene for 2 hours? Of course not.

In what seemed to be an act of anger, the district attorney then charged Billy with felony unauthorized use of a vehicle as a back up. The problem with this charge was that the only ones harmed by this action were US, and there was no way we were going to testify against Billy on this charge. We would not show up for this trial, and there would be no case.

Billy's attorney also got the trial postponed until 30 January 2007, hoping that maybe the importance of this hit and run felony trial would diminish by then.

In August, Billy managed to encounter a Loudoun County Mental Health worker who was very helpful named Sherry. Billy was required to attend meetings with Sherry twice a week as part of his probation. Sherry seemed to understand what Billy was facing and really seemed to make progress with him. She cared about her job and she wanted to make a positive difference in a life- and to this point that had been pretty rare in the "system". I was beginning to realize that only about 1 of 5 psychiatrists, probation officers, therapists, etc. would prove to actually HELP Billy with his mental illness and addictions, but unfortunately one had to wade through the 4 bad ones to get to one who really turned out to be helpful. And... we did everything we could to hang on to the helpful ones while we could- they made all the difference in saving Billy's life!

With September rolling around and no house prospects in sight, Janice had had enough of corralling Billy by herself. Although he was not drinking or drugging, he was constantly tugging at her to do this and that and craving constantly. We agreed they needed to join me in Florida if we could find someone to stay in the house while we waited for an offer to come through. I was having a very tough time renting a place that took dogs,

BILLY

and if they did they wanted a huge deposit. My housing reimbursement from Northrop Grumman was exhausted, so we would have to pay for our mortgage AND a rental. Owners would not even CONSIDER certain breeds, and honestly I was concerned that Harvey would jump the fence and attack other dogs or people. I was at the point of asking Janice to decide between staying in Virginia with the dog or coming to FL without him.

During the summer I had a chance to get back to our old church, Christian Development Center in Palm Bay, FL. This time I had a chance to play in the praise band and to my surprise there were still a lot of members there from when we left in 1995. After practice, I told our pastor Stuart Rowan and wife Terri of our dilemma, and it so happened they had a rental house available in mid September! This was truly an answer to prayer. He only wanted $900 per month, and did not demand any first, last rent or security deposit, so long as I promised to fix any damage that might be caused. We happily agreed and we were set to move in on a handshake. What a nice contrast to what we had been through in Virginia.

In mid-September I flew up to get the family so we could drive back to Florida. Janice found a nice guy, her boss's brother in law to move into the house and pay the utilities for us. We were reluctant to rent it to anyone because of our terrible experience with renters. I got there on 14 September so we could pack up and head back.

The night before we were scheduled to leave, Billy and I were sitting on the back porch chilling out. Harvey came out and immediately figured out a way to nose open the latch to the gate and take off after a neighbor walking her dog. Harvey had charged her and her dog a few weeks earlier I heard and she just stood there screaming threatening to sue. I bolted after him trying to get him to stop charging the woman, but Billy didn't move. He left me to run like a crazy man by myself screaming because he felt the lady "deserved it". The problem with that theory was that I was responsible for any damage the dog caused, not him! Harvey was fast and I kept running after him and screaming while he continually got away from me charged the lady and her dog. After 10 minutes, Janice finally heard me and drove down the street and managed to somehow get Harvey to jump in the car with her. Hoarse and furious, I went back to the house wondering why Billy didn't even attempt to help me!

Back at the house, not only was Billy NOT sorry, he was belligerent! After a few minutes he became threatening, noting all the things he would do to us if we took his dog! I heard enough and called the police. While I was calling the police, Janice took Harvey to the car and tried to drive off with him so Billy would not let the dog loose to run as he had threatened to do. Seeing Janice try to drive off, Billy became insane and jumped on the back of the PT cruiser and rode on it as Janice tried to get away. Halfway up the next street, Billy smashed the back window and leapt into the front seat where he yanked the hand brake and caused the car to skid into the ditch! Janice described it as a moment out of a Stephen King movie!

I was still at the house wondering what was going on when an officer had stopped by and told me Billy and Janice were involved in an "incident" but said nothing more. Moments later Janice came back to the house screaming and then Billy was following her on foot like nothing was wrong!

BILLY

We demanded the police arrest Billy for damage to our property, but realizing we were a day away from taking him out of THEIR hair, they resisted! One officer actually had the nerve to claim that we STOLE Billy's dog and they were going to arrest US for felony dognapping!

I was not about to be intimidated by this stupid threat. I told them that if they thought they had a case, go ahead and arrest us. They knew we were calling their bluff. Janice got the papers out for the dog and proved that SHE owned Harvey not Billy. Finally, the older officer caved and agreed that they could arrest Billy for damaging our property, but warned that would mean we would have to come back to Virginia for ANOTHER hearing. I told them I didn't care what this meant, if Billy were not arrested for this, it would mean that what he did was OK and he would go out and do some other crazy stunt and we would NEVER get to Florida. They arrested him but the magistrate released him later that night, and after asking his mother if he could come home and quietly sleep in his room, I brought him home.

From past experience, the arrest was critical. If the police walked away, he would have been unbearable to deal with and emboldened to demand whatever he wanted. Now, he was apologetic and sorry for what he had done, and realized he could have been stuck in Virginia for this stunt.

Chapter 25

Billy was very sorry the next day and wanted to come with me to have the window replaced. He vowed to pay for it first thing when we got to Florida. Also, he willingly agreed to let Harvey go- he could see we would have no room for such a wild dog in a rental house. It was hard for him, but he and Janice took Harvey to a 23 acre farm where he had all the room in the world to run.

For most people, if there son smashed the back car window and yanked the brake up on a car as it was in motion they would have nothing to do with him. I know that. But given that Billy was actually sorry of what he did and he did not look like he would cause any more problems getting down the road, we accepted his apology and hit the road.

We made it to Florida with little trouble. We soon got the keys and were guiding the movers into our rental house in southern Palm Bay, FL. Billy had really made a great effort to stop the drinking and DXM, and he seemed happy we were all together again. We took him to Dr. Vicki, his old psychiatrist from the 90s, as soon as he made it down here. We were hopeful things would go well, but we were already seeing signs of schizo-affective disorder.

When we moved into the house, we started hearing about what "Chief" wanted him to do everyday. Again, by and large they were good things- honor your parents and house, honor Mother Nature (although that made it hard to mow the grass). He also started being paranoid about germs and wearing gloves and masks all the time. He also changed out all the regular light bulbs with purple lights. He started unpacking the boxes even

BILLY

though I told him to LEAVE THEM ALONE because we were moving to another house in a few months.

Billy was getting increasingly antsy, so I took him for a canoe trip in the Indian River the next weekend. While canoeing, I told him how my OLD office got a call from his old probation officer telling a stranger that she was Billy's probation officer and she was looking to talk to me about his probation! While I felt that she had no business doing that, Billy hit the roof. It took me an hour to calm him down.

The following weekend in September we went to see the Tampa Bay Devil Rays play the Yankees. It was the first major league game Billy had ever seen. He had a great time, and in spite of a pushy seat attendant. We came back home incident free- Billy even predicted the Rays would shut out the Yankees- and they did 8-0!

I decided to continue the father-son weekend theme the next weekend and we went to a Seminole reservation south of Lake Okeechobee. We had the best time. Billy got in touch with all the Native Americans running the camp. Janice talked to her brother that weekend and found that she was part Pamunkey Indian herself. We both learned a lot. He decided to go cold turkey on his Xanax that night and I had to struggle to get him back in the car on the way home.

Staying at home during the day was doing Billy no good. He seemed to be getting stranger every day, and he was still losing weight. I helped him fill out an application for Goodwill in Melbourne, and they accepted him! He took his drug test and passed with flying colors and he started work on 15 October 2006.

It took some getting used to, but Billy actually did pretty well on his 20 hour schedule. Janice usually dropped him off and I picked him up, and usually coached him a little bit on how to handle the boredom and control his temper. Billy was a great worker- when he had down time he would clean the back of the store even while others found ways to take breaks.

On 8 November that all ended. After an hour sailing up at Cape Canaveral, I dropped Billy off at the store early. Apparently another employee aggravated him and he yelled "Get the fuck away from me". Unfortunately that was enough to get him released early that day, and when he returned the following Monday he was let go.

I felt that Billy was so close to succeeding. He had started to take his hours seriously, and doing better with his temper, and most importantly really enjoying his job. We talked every day about handling stressful situations, and it was looking like it was paying off to me. I tried to help him get the job back, but it didn't happen.

The weekend before, Billy had accidentally taken 22 Seroquel. When he started to pass out, we called the police (one of many times) and this time they rushed him to the hospital to pump his stomach. The normal dosage of Seroquel was one per day, so this was rightfully classified as a major overdose. Billy was Baker Acted immediately.

While we were waiting in the waiting room to see if Billy would make it through this overdose, Janice and I both remembered the words his last probation officer told me 10 months earlier- the next time Billy attempts to commit suicide, maybe it would be for the best to just let him die. This incensed us to the point of calling that PO and her supervisor again. Although neither had returned my

BILLY

calls before when I called about the matter, we felt like we needed to call again. We each took turns leaving messages to both of them about how we felt about that advice. As expected, we did not hear a response from either of them.

We got the good news a couple hours later that Billy was going to pull through. They took him straight to Circles of Care and really did a good job of working with him. He checked out a few days later, but surprisingly we had to then take Billy to a doctor afterwards to certify that Billy had been in the hospital in order for him to go back to work at Goodwill. A note from Circles of Care was not good enough.

We noticed a big difference between Virginia TDOs and Florida "Baker Acts". Billy was much more in control of his medications in Florida than he did when he was in Virginia. As I mentioned earlier, each of the Virginia short term TDOs brought new doctors and new medicine. Each time, the new doctor showed very little concern about what medicine or therapy Billy was on when he was admitted. The short term attitude was apparent.

In Circles of Care, the psychiatrists took time to talk with Billy before recommending anything. They also took time to talk with US- with Billy's permission of course- about what was going on. We were relieved because now we felt comfortable about Baker Acting Billy if the situation called for it.

One good thing about Billy not having a job was that he was free to go with us to the Keys over the Thanksgiving holidays. We all had a great time there, even with a few tense moments. I notice when Billy was physically active he was a lot better behaved. We got some great pictures- even one of him cutting open a coconut!

Although Billy had quit drinking, he was becoming increasingly dependent on his Ambien to sleep at night. In early December 2006, he started demanding more Ambien to sleep from our safe, and of course it was 11:30 at night. Then the threats and the cussing hit. I got out of the house long enough to call the police, only to have them come over and tell us he didn't meet criteria to be taken anywhere. Apparently the threats were not severe enough.

I paid attention when 911 begot the "terrorist threats" legislation that made it a crime to threaten terrorist action. If the same were done for threats to other family members living in the house, it would have been much easier to get Billy out of the house BEFORE he had a manic attack and caused lots of damage. As it stood now, he was a member of the household and it would take 30 days and an eviction notice to remove him from the house. IF we went through with it, then he could never come back, even if he got stable on his meds. Clearly there were no good laws to deal with the situation we constantly faced.

We got him to go to sleep that night, but Janice and I immediately went to the courthouse the next morning to ask that he be either Baker Acted for threatening us or arrested for domestic violence. While we were at the courthouse, we called for an officer to go over to the house and protect it from being destroyed! Fortunately, they sent over a Crisis Intervention Trained (CIT) officer, who handled Billy beautifully. Before this Billy was threatening to smash a policeman's face in before he was taken down, apparently this officer calmed Billy down enough to get him to call us to apologize!

BILLY

Meanwhile Janice and I filled out pages of paperwork making our request to a Judge. Unbelievably, we would not be able to go before a judge to plead our case, we had to fill out paperwork and let him take days to make a decision! I had never heard of such a ridiculous thing in my life! Sure enough, FOUR days later we get a call that Billy did not meet criteria of being a threat to himself or someone else and, since he didn't physically hit us, he didn't meet the criteria for domestic violence.

Fortunately, Billy was afraid enough to calm down, behave and go by the house rules, which is what we wanted anyway. Again, we were back to the "wait until he really does something serious before we do anything" mentality which we had seen so much of in Virginia. Obviously THIS was not going to be a realistic way of forcing Billy to get help.

The next weekend was a good one. We finally got a solid offer for $400 K on the Virginia house, and in this depressed market we took it. After looking at nearly 100 houses, we found one on Merritt Island which we really liked. It had the huge oak trees that Billy loved, it had the screened in pool and fireplace that Janice loved, and it had its own harbor for my sailboat! My initial reaction was lets think about it, but after a few minutes Billy said "Dad, this is our dream house- we have the Virginia house under contract- we really should make an offer NOW or it will be sold!" The owners were asking $595K for it, we offered them $550K and they took it. We signed the sales contract that Sunday.

We had a nice Christmas break, as our grandson Chris and stepdaughter Lisa came to visit us. During this time, I flew to Dulles to pick up the last of our belongings and then drive back. The closing went smoothly on 11

January 2007, and we were ready to move into our new house at the end of the month.

During this time period, Billy had applied for SSI benefits. I helped him with the application, which showed all 20 of his TDOs/commitments over the previous 4 years. The interview went well and we were confident he would be awarded benefits for his condition.

Billy was getting increasingly nervous about his hearing on 29 January. And he was acting stranger than ever with the face masks, purple gloves and voices in his head. On Friday 13 January Billy came home with over 100 ant bites on his hand. When we asked him what happened, he told us Chief wanted him to prove himself with a native American custom of putting his hand in a fire ant hill to show he could tolerate the pain of ant bites! I wanted to immediately call the police to have him committed, but I was fearful they would tell me he would not meet criteria and we would have called for nothing.

The next morning I had to go into work for a couple hours, and I could not get my mind off of what Billy had done. What if the next thing he did was throw himself into a fire or jump off a building? After work was done, I stopped into Circles of Care and talked to the attending counselors who told me that what Billy did should definitely meet the "hurting himself" criteria. This motivated me to stop by the Palm Bay Police office where I talked to the on duty officer. He told me that there was no doubt that letting 100 fire ants sting you met the "hurting himself" criteria. He told me if I needed to call the police today, that if any of his officers doubted that this met the criteria they need to call him immediately and he would set them straight.

BILLY

Sure enough, by that night Billy was again demanding more Ambien than he was allowed to have. He started getting loud, threatening us and walking around the house cussing. I grabbed the house phone and walked out of the house to call the police, but he had taken the phone off the hook so I could not do that. It was now 12:30 am and no one was up. How was I going to call the police? I hated leaving Janice in the house when he was manic, but someone had to get help. Besides, even when he was manic he never hurt his mother. I finally managed to find some teenagers on the next street that let me use their cell phone, but it only had 1 minute of battery time left. Fortunately I got my address of our house out along with my plea for help before the phone died.

The police showed up 5 minutes later thank goodness. He questioned Billy about the ant bites and he told him that "Chief" had told him to do this. Sure enough, after assessing the situation, the officer came to me and said "I don't know- this is kind of a borderline situation". I said "Officer, there is nothing borderline about it. By deliberately putting his hand in a fire ant hill, he endangered himself and needs to be committed. If you have a problem with that, we can call your supervisor who would be happy to help you make the proper assessment." The officer turned to Billy and said "Do you have a sweatshirt you can put on for a trip to Circles of Care?" Realizing he had little choice, Billy agreed to be voluntarily committed.

That preparation earlier that morning really paid off. Billy was taken to Circles of Care on his own terms, and while he was there, they found he had a terrible kidney infection! I knew he had felt hot for the last couple of days, but he said it was nothing he felt fine! The doctors told me this probably was a result of him wearing the skin tight leather pants day and night that caused him to hold in his urine for days at a time. They gave him antibiotics in time before the infection did any serious damage.

While there, Billy had a chance to talk to a Dr. V. He had seen clients like Billy before who became lost in the system, and although he had a full caseload, he thought he could help him. I thought we have been through 4 bad ones; we are due someone who can really help him. Billy happily agreed, and so did we. Dr. V. took our insurance, and really had a good rapport with Billy. He advocated that Billy continue to take his Seroquel and time-release Adderall as prescribed, but also was a big believer in proper nutrition. This trip to Circles of Care was really, really helpful.

As the days got closer to the hearing, Billy became increasingly fretful. I explained to Billy that I thought he had a good chance of getting a not guilty verdict in the hit-and-run charge because Billy's attorney saw to it that the prosecution could not bring up the fact that he drank anything. After all, he was away from the scene only 26 minutes and the on-site policeman described Billy as cooperative. Besides, he could not commit himself and get out of the charge. If he failed to appear for the trial, an immediate felony warrant would be issued for his arrest and he would get an additional felony charge. If he didn't go, he would just be digging himself a deeper hole. Finally, he agreed he needed to be a man and face up to the charges instead of running.

The last 2 weeks, Billy focused on getting his life going on in a positive direction. He volunteered for Habitat for Humanity every Saturday, where he did a great job. He took a test for night school at Palm Bay High and passed his test with flying colors and was signed up for

BILLY

night school to finish his senior year. Our pastor Stuart Rowan wrote a wonderful note to the court noting his positive progress over the last 5 years.

The weekend before Janice and Billy were to leave for Virginia, Billy and I took a bike ride to the end of the neighborhood we lived in, then suddenly he crossed the canal to get flowers to honor the Native American dead. He then disappeared in the woods for over an hour with the cougars and the wild boars. When darkness hit, I called Janice and the police to help search for him.

He casually showed up over an hour later, and again after 20 minutes of lobbying the police, they concluded his actions did not meet the criteria to commit him. We hoped this would be the last time we would have to go through this, and two days later he and Janice were off to face trial in Virginia.

Chapter 26

On Wednesday January 24, Janice and Billy left for Virginia at 7 am. Janice drove straight through to Virginia only stopping for gas and bathroom breaks, for if Billy decided to bolt, she wanted it to be in Virginia where they would pick him up for warrant violations immediately. If he ran and was in another state, it may be days or weeks before the local authorities would look for him, allowing him the opportunity to do some crazy desperate things. They made it to Lisa's house in Hopewell, VA by 5:30 pm. That was the fastest trip our family had ever made it between Melbourne, FL to Virginia.

The hit and run charge obviously was made because the victim pressed the district attorney level additional charges. They fined him for DUI, but obviously she wanted more. She wanted him to be convicted of a felony- any felony would do.

After visiting family, Billy went to trial the morning of 29 January with his attorney. Janice could not go because then they would be able to use her as a witness in the unauthorized use trial two days later.

The trial was over in a few hours and the verdict came down hard- one year in jail! We had been warned that even if you were away from the scene of an accident even 5 minutes you were guilty of hit and run. There would be little or no access to mental health care during that time. Apparently in Virginia, the prosecution was allowed to give the first and LAST arguments, unlike the great majority of states which the defense got the last word. Billy later told me during the District Attorney's closing argument, he made it sound like Billy was a

BILLY

chronic criminal who recklessly planned to drive to the store and run into the back of a car at 10 mph. He also showed the jury all of Billy's record for the last 5 years and implored the jury to convict the chronic criminal before them. There was little evidence that his mental illness was even considered when the jury was deliberating. All of the offenses listed were directly related to his mental illness and addictions. The attorney told me there was one juror who actually wanted to send him to prison for the year.

Even though his alcohol level could not be mentioned in court, the Mothers Against Drunk Driving (MADD) contingent in the gallery made it clear that it was an issue. Billy's attorney said the MADD badges were prominent. He had fought hard from keeping alcohol consumption from being introduced at this hit and run trial.

We were really taken back from the verdict. Billy was allowed to START to get his act together, only to be thrown in jail with no mental health care at all. To add to that, since by getting convicted for hit and run, all the other smaller charges he had gotten in years passed were all invoked. For example, they caught him in the parking lot taking his prescribed medication out of his pocket, since it was not in a bottle they seized it and took 6 months to test it to verify it was Xanax. Small things, but they all added up. Why they couldn't have made him serve these charges right after the incident in 2006 was beyond me.

After the conviction, the judge told the district attorney that if someone was going to try Billy on an unauthorized use charge with no car owner there to state any harm it was not going to be in his court. The DA dropped the charge.

While in the Loudoun jail, Billy's "good" nurse Vicki asked Janice what disease he had because he looked so gaunt. We could see how she thought that- at 6'1" he was only 137 lbs with his hair falling out. The second week in the "dungeon" Billy caught the flu from one of the other inmates, and he didn't feel like calling us as much. When I called the nurse to ask how Billy was, my answer would depend on who I caught on the phone. If Ms. Vicki did, she was happy to tell us how he was doing. If one of the other two did, they refused to tell us anything- deferring to HIPAA. I then asked how I could get a release for Billy to sign, and found out they did not know what a release was! I offered to fax one to them just like they did in the hospitals, and was told this was a jail not a hospital!

My son could be dying- and these nurses would not tell me and had no means to accept a HIPAA waiver? Frustrated, I called the on duty officer to complain- he told me the best thing to do is just avoid them and wait until the "good" nurse was on duty. Ridiculous!

Loudoun finally had finished its new jail and the era of the dungeon was almost coming to a close. But alas, despite the exponentially rising population, the new jail housed the SAME number of inmates as the old one did! So the county spent a fortune on a new jail and STILL had to ship hundreds of their inmates off to other jails at the cost of $126 per person per day! Incredible.

A week later, Billy was transferred to Charlotte Courthouse Adult Detention Center in Central Virginia. We made a trip up to see him in April and fortunately he was doing ok. Charlotte Courthouse is a little rural town and everyone there had a very "down home" manner about them, which was good for Billy. We actually got to send one book at a time to him via Walmart mail order and he actually got them to read. He started reading and it seemed like he was starting to get his aptitudes back. He was not mentioning anything about voices in his head or wanting to hurt anyone anymore. He was taking just his Seroquel and gradually getting better and gaining weight.

In May Billy had his sentencing in Loudoun County. We got another letter from our pastor written and we laid out a plan of how we could keep Billy on the right track if he released him. I wrote the judge a letter explaining how it would be better for everyone if he could be released to our custody. I pointed out how it would ALSO be better for the victim because Billy had been accepted for SSI, but he could not collect while he was in jail. Once he got his benefits, he would have the means to start reimbursing her the $3631 in restitution he had ordered. The victim could get nothing as long as he was in jail.

It did not seem to matter. The prosecutor represented the victim and acted like being run into the back of at 10 mph at a stop light devastated her life forever. She didn't know if she would ever get over it because it had traumatized her that badly, the prosecutor said. It is a good thing she was not sideswiped. Don't get me wrong- this whole incident never should have happened. The victim deserves to be reimbursed for her expenses resulting from the accident. But how imprisoning someone with a mental illness for a year on a felony charge was going to solve anything was beyond me.

The judge upheld the 1 year sentence, and was considering the prosecutor's recommendation of 2 years of in-state probation. The problem was WE had moved to Florida and Florida did not have a probation exchange agreement with Virginia. To serve his 2 year probation, Billy would have to stay somehow in Virginia by himself for 2 years, or one of us would have to move BACK to Virginia and get a place so he could serve probation. Again, this part of the order seemed absolutely ludicrous to me.

The judge also ordered Billy to be re-evaluated by Loudoun County Mental Health (again- for what purpose I have not a clue) and recommend a "get well" plan for Billy. As I recall, LCMH told us the year before that they were not able to diagnose Billy.

Fortunately, at the follow-up hearing, there was a substitute judge on the bench. After hearing Billy's story, he saw no point in giving him probation in Virginia when he had no home in Virginia. Instead, his 6 month probation would consist of getting reports from Dr. V once a month for 6 months. Sometimes justice came in the form of a lucky break- like a judge not being on the bench on a follow-up hearing day.

The biggest challenge we faced while Billy was at Charlotte Courthouse ADC was keeping his supply of Seroquel. Even though Billy made requests when the supply was about to run out, it would always become a crisis when he had only days worth of medication left and no refill was on the way. Billy at this stage in his life understood how important it was to take his medication properly, and the last thing he wanted to do is go manic in jail and get more charges. Conceivably he could stay in jail the rest of his life before someone figured it out.

In the early days, we had to scramble to get his medication refilled in a timely manner. Janice figured out who his local doctor was, Dr. Wayland, and called his office directly. Usually he managed to go over and see Billy right away, and acted as his advocate in getting his meds to him before the last pill ran out. Even

BILLY

the sheriff told us HE would go to the pharmacy personally if he needed to.

One month he got down to one pill. I faxed Dr. Wayland with Billy's prescription, I got no response. I tried calling his office, he was not in. I didn't know what else I could do without angering the jail staff, so Janice thought to mail him a personal handwritten note to him pleading for him to make sure Billy's prescription was filled. Surprisingly, it turned out to be the difference maker. The day Dr. Wayland got the note he immediately filled Billy's prescription personally and got him his medication without allowing him to miss a day. God bless him- and my wife too for writing a personal note. Never underestimate the power of a mother's heartfelt plea.

We made a point to visit Billy every 2 months or so, and fortunately he was getting better each time we saw him. His hair was coming back thick and healthy, his eyes and skin were clear. He continued to gain weight, and he was actually filling out his 6 foot frame. He would tell us he was not eligible for work release because he was a Loudoun inmate, and at the time the jail was struggling to get a GED program. When they finally got a GED training program, Billy signed up. Unfortunately, the teacher was not qualified to actually GIVE the test, so whoever signed up would have to wait until they got out to take the test. Another "are you kidding me" moment...

I could not help but think during this time- what a waste of a year. Yes he was convicted of hit and run, but why exacerbate that by giving him nothing to do for a year? Again we heard that the jail did not have much money, and we made sure he had enough canteen money to get plenty of snacks to supplement the meals.

So here is where we ended up. For years we tried to get help for Billy and his bipolar disorder, and we were told that the best thing to do was let him go manic and commit a crime and once arrested, we could then get help for him. But when that happens, he is treated like a common criminal and sent to a place for a year with no mental health care. Once that verdict is read, no one cares that he is someone with a mental health problem, he is just another inmate.

Not only is mental health care not available, regular medical care is iffy too. Billy told us about an inmate who decided to arm wrestle and actually broke his arm. The jail had no money to have a doctor treat him, so they just wrapped his arm up without setting it! I think they treat people on the street better than this!

In January 2008 we got word that Charlotte Courthouse ADC could not afford to pay for Billy's medication anymore, and they asked Loudoun County to pay. I had talked to the new head of LCMH, Tom Maynard, a few months earlier about what I thought could be done to improve things for the clients of Loudoun County. He had assigned a staff member to monitor Billy's progress, and Loudoun County immediately agreed to pay for Billy's Seroquel. We were all very grateful.

As Billy's term comes to a close on 4 April, there were a few twists. Out of the blue, Billy was called up to Loudoun for a hearing 7 March 2008. Apparently the district attorney accusing him of failing to complete his probation conditions in February 2007 by failing to meet with his psychiatrist Dr. V. The problem was- he was in JAIL in February 2007. Luckily they were able to reach Billy's attorney who had to actually show papers to the new judge that Billy was in Loudoun jail during this time. When the presiding judge heard this, she asked why on

BILLY

earth would the prosecutor waste her time with this charge. In the same hearing though, they had established Billy had no violations whatsoever and would get all his good time applied. We were so glad the Seroquel had worked so well this time and indeed Billy was going to be out of that system forever.

Before he got out, he was transferred to Middle River ADC. Amazingly, they put him in solitary because he had kicked out the windows in a police cruiser in 2002 when he was clearly manic. Even though he had been an angel for a year, this is what they went by. I guess the fact that the Loudoun police completely dropped the charge in 2002 when Billy agreed to get help was irrelevant.

Postlude

As with life, there are no guarantees when you have a child that he or she will be totally healthy. No one ever asks to have a bipolar child. However, if one is to be a good parent, they take the good with the bad and try to do what they can to make the best life they can for that child.

Obviously a mental illness is something no one wants to have. Billy certainly didn't want it, but he got it. He got the phenomenal craving for drugs that many times accompanies this condition. When his "rights" to not take his medication or to become manic were granted to him, believe me he is not feeling patriotic about it. Billy will tell you now that those are rights he would gladly have given up if it would have allowed us to keep him from getting into trouble. In fact, he would have been happy to give those rights back for a normal life any day.

After this happened, long term care for mental illness all but disappeared. This didn't fix any problems, however, the problems created from this change in philosophy still had to be addressed. Those problems fell on law enforcement whether they wanted to deal with them or not.

Trying to solve long term chronic solutions with 3 day stays does not work either. Chronic long term solutions need long term care. Law enforcement has in place progressively more severe penalties for persons who commit repeat offenses, yet mental health is stuck with a single 3 day "band aid" solution no matter how many times a patient is committed. And continuing to put band-aids on gaping wounds just promotes infection.

BILLY

In general, law enforcement will not "anticipate" the results of a manic incident. Even though we have seen a dangerous situation develop time and time again, no one will react until he actually attempts to hurt himself or others. We can anticipate the actions of terrorists, but we cannot do this for persons with mental illness.

Further, since law enforcement has been forced to deal with the problem of mental illness, EVERY police unit should get CIT trained so they can properly deal with our loved ones. Freezing parents out of helping their kids is just the wrong thing to do. It hurts the mentally ill kids, it hurts the innocent people encounter a manic client, and it hurts society because they have to pay for improperly detaining them.

Who had the bright idea to incarcerate the chronically mentally ill anyway? From what I could see, mental health therapy ceases once someone is incarcerated. Encouraging family members to "let" persons with mental illness commit crimes so they can get "services" is just wrong, just as wrong as encouraging families to evict mentally-affected members from their household and let them "sink or swim" on the streets. Without the right medication and backup from family/friends, the great majority will sink, often doing terrible harm to innocent people. If a client has become stable, incarcerating them with no mental health care may trigger them to be manic more often and could trigger and unnecessary endless stream of violations in which the client will never get out of jail – and never get the right help.

Persons with mental illness in general are not criminals. Billy is not a criminal, yet he was saddled with a felony because of a manic incident. He has a family that loves him and will do anything to help him get better. Yet all these resources did not stop any of the events that happened.

For us, God has allowed us to have our son back despite all odds. He did not crack after being stuck in jail for over a year as he could have. Many parents in our same situation have not been as fortunate, and this many times have left us wondering "why us"? We are incredibly thankful for that, and I have said many times I would give up anything that I have gained over life to have a "normal" son, a son that has control over his life. It looks to me like despite everything everyone has been through, we just may get that.

Billy is getting social security starting in April 2008, and he is welcome to stay with us as long as he would like. I was encouraged to see him now dare to dream. Dream to one day get married and have children. Dream to have a job and place of his own someday. And dream to have a life of his own. He deserves it.

www.ingramcontent.com/pod-product-compliance
Ingram Content Group UK Ltd.
Pitfield, Milton Keynes, MK11 3LW, UK
UKHW041411180426
11947UKWH00007B/57